Clinical Capillaroscopy

With compliments **SCHERING**

Alfred Bollinger
Bengt Fagrell

Clinical Capillaroscopy

A Guide to Its Use in Clinical Research and Practice

Hogrefe & Huber Publishers
Toronto • Lewiston, NY • Bern • Göttingen • Stuttgart

Canadian Cataloguing in Publication Data

Main entry under title:
Clinical capillaroscopy

1. Capillaries—Examination. 2. Capillaries—Diseases—Diagnosis. 3. Microcirculation.
4. Microscopy, Medical. I. Bollinger, A. (Alfred), 1932—   . II. Fagrell, Bengt.

QP106.6.C58   1990   616.1'48   C90-094817-5

No part of this book may be reproduced, stored in a retrieval system, or transmitted, in any form or by any means, electronic, mechanical, photocopying, microfilming, recording or otherwise, without written permission from the publisher.

© Copyright 1990 by Hogrefe & Huber Publishers

P. O. Box 51
Lewiston, NY 14092

12–14 Bruce Park Ave.
Toronto, Ontario M4P 2S3

ISBN 3-456-81924-2
ISBN 0-88937-048-6
Hogrefe & Huber Publishers • Toronto • Lewiston, NY • Bern • Göttingen • Stuttgart

Printed in Germany

Table of Contents

Foreword vii
    Historical Overview   vii
    Modern Clinical Microcirculation   viii
    Aims of the Book and Acknowledgments   ix

1 TECHNIQUES AND NORMAL FINDINGS 1
    1.1 Ordinary Capillaroscopy   1
    1.2 Dynamic Capillaroscopy Without Dyes   9
    1.3 Dynamic Capillaroscopy with Dyes (Fluorescence Video Microscopy)   31
    1.4 Fluorescence Microlymphography   53
    1.5 Combination of Techniques   60

2 PATHOLOGICAL CONDITIONS 63
    2.1 Arterial Occlusive Disease (Ischemia)   63
    2.2 Diabetes   77
    2.3 Chronic Venous Incompetence (CVI)   93
    2.4 Lymphedema   107
    2.5 Vasospastic Diseases   115
    2.6 Collagen Vascular Disease and Related Disorders   121
    2.7 Hematological Disorders   144
    2.8 Miscellaneous Disorders   147

3 CONTROL OF THERAPY 155
    3.1 Pharmacological Agents   155
    3.2 Interventional Therapy   159

Subject Index 163

FOREWORD

Historical Overview

In his famous work *De motu cordis et sanguinis* (1628), William Harvey described for the first time the blood circulation without discovering the capillaries. Only in 1661 did Marcello Malpighi recognize the tiny vessels linking the arterial and venous system. Soon afterwards Antony van Leeuwenhoeck observed the blood cells moving in frog capillaries. John Marshall, a grinder of lenses and constructor of microscopes, observed the circulating blood in the microcirculation of a fish tail around 1700. The optical system was illuminated by a burning candle (see **Figure** below).

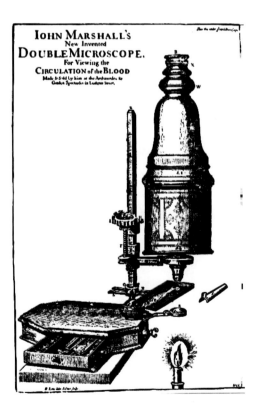

During the following century, no major progress was made. In 1831, Marshall Hall distinguished precapillary, capillary, and postcapillary vessels. Among the first he ranged vessels still ramifying downstream, among the latter those merging to larger trunks—a definition that is still accepted today.

A more sophisticated view was gained around the turn of the century by Frank Starling, who established his famous, and still controversial, equation about capillary exchange of fluid and solutes. But it was the studies carried out by August and Marie Krogh that opened the way to modern microvascular physiology. They described the diffusion of oxygen through the wall of microvessels and showed that the number of perfused muscle capillaries varies according to the state of muscular activity. In 1920, August Krogh received the Nobel Prize for his achievements.

The pioneer time for clinical microcirculation was between the two world wars. The astonishing work performed by Otfried Müller in Tübingen was dedicated to capillaroscopy through intact human skin. Since microphotography was not yet developed, the capillaries were drawn in color by expert artists. It is still a challenging pleasure to leaf through his book *Die Kapillaren der menschlichen Körperoberfläche in gesunden und kranken Tagen* (1922). His images, demonstrating even the movement of plasma gaps in nailfold capillary loops, fascinated pupils like Walter Redisch, who today at over 90 years lives in New York City and follows the developments in clinical microcirculation with great interest. Human capillary physiology had its first milestone during the same period when Eugene Landis measured nailfold capillary pressure (1930).

In the late 1950s and the early 1960s, a movement took place that Paul Johnson from Tucson, Arizona, called the "Renaissance of microcirculation." La Jolla in Southern California became a center of particular importance because of the outstanding and stimulating work performed by Benjamin Zweifach and his group. This period was characterized by rapid development of television techniques, which facilitated enormously the task of analyzing dynamic events in the microcirculation.

Bioengineers made decisive advances in developing techniques suited for modern research. Marcos Intaglietta and Curt Wiederhielm built micropressure systems and video densitometers; Harold Wayland's intravital microscope was two stories high; and Max Anliker's "blue elephant" was equipped with two television cameras operating with an adjustable time delay.

Modern Clinical Microcirculation

In clinical microcirculation, the books published by Davis and Landau as well as by Illig maintained the interest during the 1960s. The 1970s started with Brånemark's important monograph entitled *Intravascular Anatomy of Blood Cells in Man*. Whereas the latter publication was based on capsules implanted by surgical means, Hildegard Maricq and the authors tried to introduce more sophisticated techniques for conventional capillaroscopy and systems for analyzing dynamic phenomena. First, blood cell velocity was measured in human skin capillaries. Some years later, transcapillary and interstitial diffusion of sodium fluorescein was assessed by fluorescence video microscopy and video densitometry. During the 1980s, it became possible to stain and visualize lymphatic microvascular networks and to introduce indocyanine green as a second fluorescent tracer useful for detailed studies. The determination of blood cell velocity was automatized by novel procedures based on computer-aided densitometry and image analysis.

Two other techniques have enriched the armamentarium of the clinical microcirculationist: laser Doppler and transcutaneous measurement of oxygen pressure. Flux in nonnutritional shunt vessels dominates the signal recorded by the laser Doppler, while transcutaneous oxygen pressure most probably reflects primarily the function of the nutritive skin capillaries. The only method that evaluates blood flow in the nutritional capillaries with certainty is capillaroscopy. As only a minute (<15%) part of the skin microcirculation passes these capillaries (see **Figure** below), capillaroscopy is the best choice for studying the nutritional status of a certain skin area.

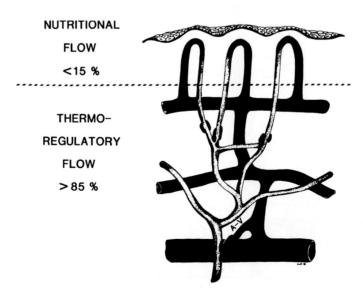

Foreword

First comparisons between capillaroscopic findings and the two other methods have been published. At present, attempts are being made to combine the different approaches, for example, by the so-called triple probe, which has a translucent central part with a miniaturized oxygen electrode melted into the glass cylinder and optical fibers leading the laser light through the outer ring of the probe containing heating elements.

Aims of the Book and Acknowledgments

A considerable part of the book is dedicated to the techniques now available in clinical capillaroscopy. Details on our own work are provided. The text includes the conventional procedure and the sophisticated methods for measurement of blood cell velocity and transcapillary diffusion of small fluorescent molecules. How to depict the plasma layer by indocyanine green and to color microlymphatics is also described.

In contrast to the laser Doppler and the transcutaneous oxygen pressure measurements, which have already been subject of comprehensive monographs or articles, modern capillaroscopy has yet to be presented in a textbook form. Observation of capillaries through the intact human skin provides direct information on dynamic events occurring in this important part of the circulation not available by indirect techniques.

In a number of chapters the data obtained thus far by the different approaches are presented in various disease states. An astonishing amount of information has been accumulated over the last few years concerning as different conditions as ischemia, diabetes, chronic venous insufficiency, lymphedema, and Raynaud's phenomenon. These available data now form a basis for application in clinical medicine and for future research. The world of clinical microcirculation is still largely unexplored.

Microangiopathies are important per se in diabetes and collagen vascular disease. In other conditions, like the broad spectrum of ischemic diseases and chronic venous incompetence, microvascular morphology and function are disturbed as a consequence of macrovascular damage. Microcirculation is the target section under both circumstances: The changes at this level decide whether a tissue survives or dies.

The techniques described may also be used to quantify drug effects at the microvascular level. Statements to the effect that "a medicament probably influences microcirculation" because there is no better explanation, are no longer valid. The methods to prove such a statement are established and should be used to solve these problems.

The authors are indebted to their friends working in microcirculation. Their input from basic and clinical science, their criticism and encouragement were crucial in the writing of this book. Special thanks go to the young colleagues who work or have worked in our laboratories, who have contributed to the accumulation of valid data, and who have stimulated us through their enthusiasm. Yes, there are still fundamental phenomena to be discovered in clinical microcirculation!

The work performed would not have been possible without the generous support from our department chairmen. In particular, the authors thank Professor Walter Siegenthaler and Professor Göran Holm. We are indebted to the technicians Mirjam Geiger, Barbara Dubler, and Ann-Christin Salomonsson, who contributed enormously to the success of many studies performed in our laboratories.

Most gratefully we acknowledge the financial support provided by the Kanton of Zürich, the Karolinska Institute, the Swiss National Science Foundation, the Bonizzi-Theler Foundation, the Swedish Medical Research Council and the Swedish Heart and Lung Foundation. Without their substantial help over many years this textbook would never have appeared.

1

TECHNIQUES AND NORMAL FINDINGS

1.1 Ordinary Capillaroscopy

Microscope

The skin capillaries can be studied directly with an ordinary light, preferably stereo, microscope with a total magnification from 10–100× (11, 12, 15, 23*). The microscope most often used in clinical practice today is the Wild-Leitz 3M® Stereo Microscope, with a possible magnification from 10 up to 100× (**Figure 1**).

If an overview of all the nailfold capillaries is wanted, a widefield system should be used. A photomacrography system has been developed by Maricq (45, 46), the system being composed of a Topcon Super DM camera body, Model IV bellows, and a Macro Auto-Topcor lens (**Figure 2**). This set up gives an overview of about 6–8 mm and makes it very easy to do morphology analyses of the capillaries.

* The numbers refer to the respective reference sections at the end of each chapter.

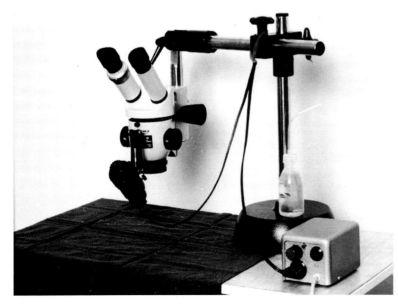

Figure 1. Equipment for vital capillaroscopy. The microscope is a Wild-Leitz 3M® stereomicroscope with variable magnification from 10 to 40×.

1

Chapter 1.1

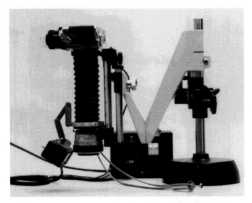

Figure 2. Equipment for widefield photography of skin capillaries. (With permission from 46)

Suspension of the Microscope

Since small movements and vibrations of the microscope would interfere with the observations, the microscope should be mounted on a firm stand. The stand should include a movable arm so that the whole equipment can be moved in any direction (**Figure 1**).

Magnification

For morphological studies a magnification from about 5–100× is appropriate. This is the magnification the microscope itself gives. However, nowadays a combination of a microscope and a television setup is often used, so that the magnification varies with the size of the monitor (see also below "Dynamic Capillaroscopy Without Dyes").

Illumination

In the Wild-Leitz 3M system, the skin surface is illuminated by an AC-powered 15 W microscope lamp that can be moved in any direction around the center of the area under observation. This makes it possible to adjust the direction of the light in order to avoid disturbing reflections from the skin surface, which should be illuminated at an angle of approximately 45° for optimal view. The light should be focused on an area of approximately 1 cm^2.

In order to make the skin transparent and to further minimize the reflections from the skin surface, some kind of oil has to be applied to the skin. Least expensive is paraffin oil, which is also easily accessible in the hospital.

The Skin Surface

In all subjects with a normal peripheral circulation, the skin surface is relatively transparent, making the apical part of the capillaries easily visible for direct study. In some patients, the skin surface may be less transparent, possibly because of structural changes in the epidermis itself or because of the presence of interfering substances on the surface of the skin. In these cases, the horny layer may have to be removed. This can be done by peeling off the horny layer with the sharp end of an injection needle so that the papillary layer is exposed. Sometimes ordinary adhesive tape can also be applied to the skin and removed several times, thus peeling off the most superficial part of the horny layer.

Filters

For optimal contrast between the capillaries and the surrounding tissue, a blue filter should be placed in front of the lamp. An additional heat-absorbing filter may also be used, but this is not necessary with a 15 W lamp. Sometimes—depending on the light source—a green filter may give a better contrast between the blood cells in the capillaries and the surrounding tissue.

Photographic or Video Recording

The microscopical observations can be recorded on ordinary photographs, but nowadays video tape is preferred. The connection between the microscope and the video or photo camera must be specified for each equipment. It should be stressed that the documentation should be made in black and white in order to achieve the best contrast between the blood-filled capillaries and the surrounding skin tissue. If color film is used, it is often difficult to get maximum contrast in the picture, and the capillaries become indistinct.

Investigating Procedure

Hands

The nailfold of the fingers has been used extensively for studying morphological changes of skin capillaries in different systemic diseases (see the individual chapters in this volume). The hand is placed on the investigation table, and a small wedge (**Figure 3**) is positioned between the object and the table in order to get the dorsal surface of the observed area in a horizontal position.

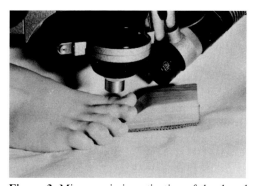

Figure 3. Microscopic investigation of the dorsal skin of the foot and toes. Notice the wooden wedge that is used for getting the skin surface horizontal.

Feet

When the feet are going to be investigated, the patient should be in a sitting position, to ensure a good blood filling of the region even in patients with markedly reduced arterial circulation of the leg (**Figure 4**). The small wedge should also be used here in order to get the skin surface under observation in a horizontal position. As always, paraffin oil should be applied to the skin surface.

Other Parts of the Body

Almost all parts of the skin surface have been studied by vital capillaroscopy. Some of these are the *bulbar conjunctiva, lip, gingiva,* and the *tongue*. The bulbar conjunctiva has been a favorite observation site for many observers since studies can be easily performed with an eye microscope or slit-lamp. The advantage of using the conjunctiva is that it is easily accessible and gives a very clear view of the network of small arterioles, capillaries, and venules. Because of the optimal contrast between the red blood cells and the surrounding white conjunctiva, it is an excellent area for clinical studies, for example, of intravascular red cell aggregation. However, movement artefacts makes it almost impossible to get good recordings of the blood flow in the

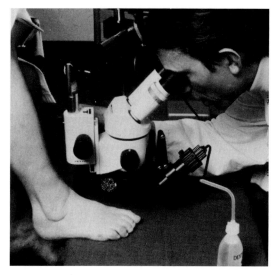

Figure 4. Investigation of the dorsal skin of the foot of a patient with PAOD and suspected skin ischemia. The patient should be investigated in a sitting position to ensure good blood filling of the microvascular bed of the area.

vessels. Ordinary black-and-white photos have to be used (11).

The capillaries of the *lower leg* have also been extensively studied, especially in patients with dermatological disorders and venous insufficiency (14, 26, 27). While the capillaries of the lower leg are being investigated, the patient should be in a supine position, and in order to ensure a good blood filling of the vascular bed of the region, a blood pressure cuff may be applied around the leg above or below the knee and inflated to a pressure of 30–60 mmHg.

Morphology Analysis

Already in 1879 Heuter presented the first study on microscopic examinations of capillaries in humans (28). He described the capillary structure of of the border of the human lip. In 1917, Weiss and Müller (61) introduced the technique as a clinical method, and in 1937 and 1939 Müller (48) published two volumes on the anatomy, physiology, and pathology of the small vessels in human skin. After this, a considerable number of studies were published on microscopic examination of the skin capillaries. Most of them are concerned with the nailfold of fingers. Some studies have also been performed in dermatological practice in skin areas affected by dermatological diseases.

Normal Patterns

— Nailfold Capillaries

As most of the studies have used the nailfold area for observation, the capillary structure in this region will be described in more detail.

The pattern of the nailfold vascular bed has been studied on postmortem specimens of human fingers by injecting a colored latex, or liquid plastic, solution followed by corrosion of the soft tissue (8, 9, 30). In most areas of the fingers the nutritional capillary loops are located in a 90° angle to the skin surface (**Figure 5**), and only the tip of the capillary loops can be visualized. Usually, there are 1–3 capillaries in each dermal papilla. In the nailfold

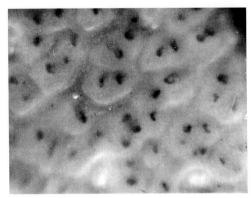

Figure 5. Microphoto of the nutritional skin capillaries of the dorsum of a finger in a healthy subject. Only the apex of the capillaries are seen as points or commas in the papillae.

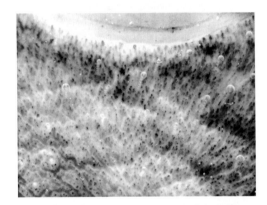

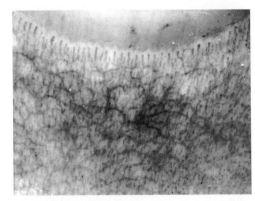

Figure 6. Widefield photos of finger nailfold capillaries in the normal subject. (Reprinted with permission from Maricq and Maize, *Clin. reum. Dis.* 8, 456, 1982.)

Table 1. Average diameters (means ± SD) of the erythrocyte column and the inside of the nailfold capillaries in 33 healthy subjects (after Mahler et al., 44).

	Erythrocyte column (a) µm	Cap. inner diameter (b) µm	b − a µm
Arteriolar limb	10.8 ± 3.0	15.0 ± 2.5	4.2 ± 0.7***
(range)	6.2–19.0	9.8–20.5	2.8–5.6
Venular limb	12.1 ± 2.7	16.7 ± 3.0	4.6 ± 0.8***
(range)	8.0–20.1	10.3–23.1	3.0–6.2

*** p<0.001

area, the capillary loops become successively more parallel to the skin surface, and in the last row they can be visualized rather nicely in their full length (**Figure 6**). Normally, the subpapillary vascular plexus cannot be seen in the nailfold, but in about 30% of healthy individuals it is visible (30, 45). The capillaries are built up by an arterial and a venous limb, and in between these two is the apical part. The arterial portion of the capillary is regularly more narrow then the venous one. The ratio of the veno/arterial diameter is approximately 1.2 to 1.5×, and there is a successive increase in diameter from the proximal, arterial side to the distal venous side. The average diameter of the arteriolar limb is 11 ± 3µm with a range from 6–19 µm, while the venular limb is 12 ± 3 µm and the range 8–20 µm (44). It should also be stressed that these diameters represent the diameter of the erythrocyte column and not the true capillary diameter, as the capillary walls can vary seldom be identified by ordinary light microscopy. By employing fluorescein isothiocyanat-human albumin (FITC-HA), the true inner diameter of the capillary can be measured. As seen in **Table 1** (44), the inner diameter of the capillaries is approximately 4–4.5 µm wider then the erythrocyte column.

The morphological pattern of the capillaries in the same finger of an individual is surprisingly constant. The structure of a specific capillary can be observed for years with the same morphological appearance (30). With age the capillaries might become slightly more tortuous and also somewhat dilated. The nailfold capillaries can be classified according to their morphology and distribution, and different classification systems have been used. One such schedule is presented in **Figure 7** (30). Some capillaries in normal subjects may have a certain degree of tortuosity in the limb, especially on the venous side. The number of visible capillaries in the nailfold range from 10 to 30 per mm^2.

— **Capillaries of the Dorsum of Hands and Feet**

Many patients with various diseases, for example, peripheral arterial insufficiency, Raynaud's phenomenon, and polycythemia, have disturbed nutritional circulation in fingers and toes. In many of these patients the structure of the nutritional skin capillaries are markedly changed, and therefore it is important to know the normal structure of the capillaries in these areas (8, 12, 16). A specific and systematic classification of the nutritional capillaries in the dorsum of the foot has been described by Fagrell in 1973 (13).

Normal structure: The capillaries have a uniform appearance in healthy subjects, irrespective of age and sex (**Figure 8**; **Table 2**). Most of the papillas are clearly outlined, and 1 to 3 capillaries are seen as dots or commas in each papilla. The capillary density of the forefoot varies from approximately 70 per mm^2 on the dorsal skin of the toes to about 30–50 per mm^2 on the foot. There is a normal tonicity in the capillary bed—a permanent variation in the diameter of the visible capillaries—within the skin area studied. Age does not seem to significantly influence capillary morphology (Ta-

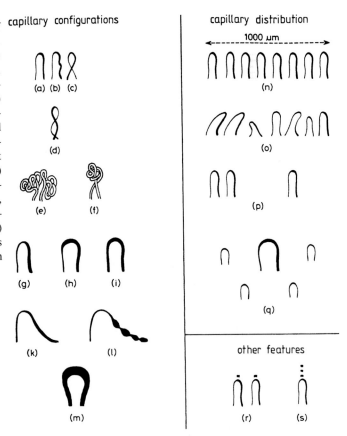

Figure 7. Different patterns of nailfold capillary morphology. *Capillary configuration:* (a)–(c) hairpin-shaped capillary loops, (d) tortuous loops, (e) bushy appearance, (f) coiled, ball, (g)–(i) enlargements of loops in the efferent, apical, and afferent and efferent part, (k)–(l) enlargements of venules, (m) giant loop. *Capillary distribution:* (n) regular distribution, (o) disarranged loops, (p) local paucity, (q) enlarged loop bordering local paucity. *Other features:* (r) extravasates, (s) pearl necklaces of extravasates. (Reprinted with permission from 30.)

Table 2. Differences between young (a), middle-aged (b), and elderly (c) normal subjects concerning the capillary structure of the dorsal skin of the toes and forefoot. The significance of difference (Mann-Whitney U-test) between the groups are given.

Group	n	Capillary stage		
		0	1	2
a (20–39 yrs)	15	20	10	0
b (40–59 yrs)	15	19	11	0
c (60–79 yrs)	15	6	16	8

a:b = p>0.05; b:c = p<0.01; a:c = p<0.01

ble 2), except for the mentioned apical dilatation of the capillaries ("micropools"), which can be found in approximately 25% of elderly, but not in young or middle age subjects (13, 54). As the subjects with micropools are quite elderly (70–79 years), it is possible that changes are present in the microcirculation of the skin, although the arterial circulation, as evaluated by digital arterial blood pressure measurements, is completely normal. Ryan and Curban (57) also found an increased tendency toward aneurysmatic dilatation of the capillaries in elderly subjects, but they did not relate their findings to the arterial circulation of the region.

Several authors have found micropools in the conjunctival vessels of healthy persons. The incidence has been reported to be 10–15% (10, 11, 47). However, Heisig did not find any micropools in 150 young individuals, but in 40% of patients with generalized arteriosclerosis (29). Aneurysmatic changes of the skin capillaries have also been observed in patients with pigmented purpuric diseases (10, 56) and cold sensitivity disorders (56).

Ordinary Capillaroscopy

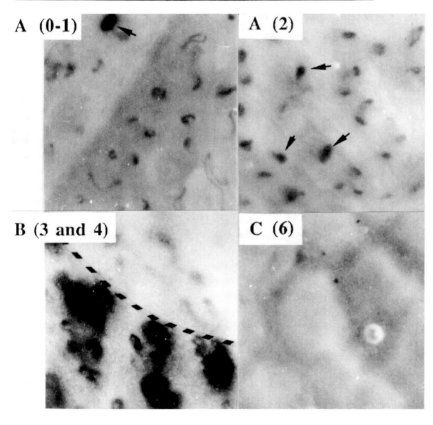

Figure 8. Classification of capillary morphology according to Fagrell (13).

* Risk of developing a skin ulcer within 3 months in the area in which the capillary stage was seen at the first observation.

STAGE	DESCRIPTION OF CHANGES	RISK OF * NECROSIS
0 (A)	Dot or comma shaped with good 'tonicity'	5 %
1 (A)	As in Stage 0, but less 'tonicity'	5 %
2 (A)	Marked dilatation and sometimes 'micropools'	5 %
3 (B)	Indistinct capillaries (e.g. edema, sclerosis)	15 %
4 (B)	Capillary hemorrhages	15 %
5 (C)	Only a few (<10) capillaries visible	90 %
6 (C)	No capillaries visible	95 %

— Lower Leg

Another area in which it is of interest to study the morphology of the nutritional skin capillaries is the distal part of the lower leg. The reason for this is that in patients with venous insufficiency microvascular disturbances is often located at the medial side of the lower leg, with hyperpigmentation, eczema, and leg ulcers (14, 55, 56). Normally, capillaries in this area are also point or comma shaped (**Figure 9**), but the number per mm^2 is only about 20–30, which is about half that of fingers and toes. Sometimes a longer portion of the capillary limbs can be visualized, especially in elderly subjects (**Figure 10**). The papillas may also be surrounded by a weak, pigmented network, especially in sun-tanned skin areas.

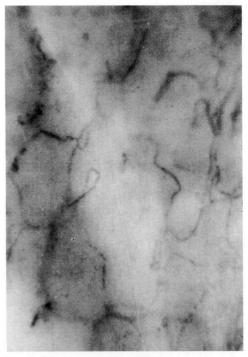

Figure 10. Skin capillaries of the lower leg of a 78-year-old woman with normal peripheral macrocirculation. Skin atrophy is present, making more of the capillary network visible.

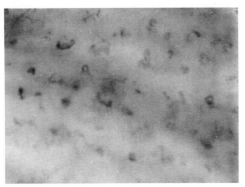

Figure 9. Nutritional capillary loops of the medial part of the lower leg in a subject with normal peripheral circulation.

— Lip, Tongue, Gingiva, and Conjunctiva

These areas are nowadays seldom studied in clinical practice by capillaroscopy. For those interested in the capillary structure of these areas, the book by Davis and Landau can be highly recommended (11).

1.2 Dynamic Capillaroscopy Without Dyes

Already in 1912 Lombard showed that it was possible to study physiological phenomena in the nailfold capillaries of humans (42). In 1919 Basler described a sophisticated mechanical set up for actual measurements of the velocity of the blood cells in human nailfold capillaries (1), and it was later shown that his measurements were surprisingly correct. In 1964, Zimmer and Demis demonstrated that it was possible to study dynamic flow properties directly, and noninvasively, in human skin capillaries by a microscope-television system (62). At about the same time, Brånemark (1964) presented an invasive technique for studying the dynamics of human skin microcirculation (4): He inserted a modified titanium chamber in a skin tube of the upper arm and was able to do pioneering, high-resolution studies on microvascular blood flow in this artificially produced scar tissue of the skin (4, 5, 52).

A new microscope-television system was introduced by Bollinger et al. in 1974 (2), and for the first time it was shown that the technique of dynamic capillaroscopy could be used clinically for studying capillary dynamics in health and disease. Fagrell et al. (1977) improved, and simplified, the technique so that it could be used in clinical practice (17, 18, 19). They also incorporated a technique for simultaneous recordings of systemic parameters, such as arterial pulsations or respiration on the video recordings (17).

Technique for Measuring Capillary Blood Cell Velocity

Analysis of *capillary blood cell velocity* (CBV) was initially performed only by observing the movements of cells and plasma gaps by the naked eye. However, already in 1919 Basler (1) described a sophisticated, mechanical setup for CBV measurements. In 1974, Bollinger et al. adapted a frame-to-frame analysis to calculate the CBV by watching the successive movements along the capillary length of plasma gaps between red cell aggregates (2). This technique is extremely time consuming and cannot follow fast dynamic changes in CBV. Fagrell et al. applied the video-photometric, cross-correlation technique of Intaglietta and coworkers (31, 32, 33) for measuring CBV in the humans skin. This technique made it possible to record CBV both continuously and accurately for long time periods (17, 18, 19). The dynamic changes of CBV could now also be studied, but a rather advanced technical skill was needed to make the system work in clinical practice. This drawback was overcome in 1988 when Fagrell et al. introduced a completely computerized system for the whole process of analysis (24). By using a sophisticated computer program, the whole process of CBV calculations can now be handled also by technically nontrained persons.

Microscope

In order to be able to measure capillary blood cell velocity (CBV) with any technique, an optimal image of the skin capillaries has to be achieved. Several kind of microscope systems have been used for this purpose. However, it is not possible to make theoretical calculations of how such a system should be composed. The combination of microscope, light source, filters, and specification of the television tube is crucial. For optimal contrast between the red blood cells in the capillary and the surrounding tissue, a certain light source will need a specific filter. One setup may work with a blue filter, while a green filter will be optimal in another system. It is therefore absolutely necessary to follow the detailed instructions given in this book for putting the different systems together. The system described in detail in this chapter has been used with great success in routine clinical practice, for measuring all kind of capillary flow dynamics in humans.

Table 3. Microscope, television camera, and monitor equipment for CBV measurements. The equipment recommended below has been thouroughly tested for studying CBV in humans. Other combination of appartus may also work nicely, but it is hazardous to buy any other equipment without testing it carefully beforehand.

MICROSCOPE	PART NO.
Microscope Leitz Laborlux 12 ME D	224.562-212
Table	224.512-695
Tube	224.512-736
Lamp body 103 Z	224.514-687
Collector	224.514-727
Lamp-holder IREM-HIBN/Hg 100	224.620-806
Hg-Lamp 100W	224.700-138
IR-filter	224.514-710
Stabilized aggregate IREM-EB-XH 5 P/L	224.620-801
1-lambda-pleumopak (TL 1×), Bg 38	224.513-591
Filter system-POL	224.502-509
Objective PL 2.5/0.08	224.519-495
Objective PL FLUOTAR 10/0.30	224.519-872
Objective NPL FLUOTAR L 25/0.30	224.519-679
C-adapter for camera 0.1×*	224.543-513
Clamping sleeve	224.543-352
Tube, Wild TL160	224.445-091
Ocular PERIPLAN GF 12, 5×/20, photo, TL 160	224.519-881
Finger holder	IM CapiFlow

VIDEO CAMERA
Hitachi HV-725E or
Ikegami CTC-2110 with silicon diode tube RCA 4532
New, so-called CCD cameras are also available, but the contrast is sometimes much less than in tube cameras, and consequently they must be tested thoroughly before being purchased.

VIDEO MONITOR
Hitachi VM 920 or
Ikegami 5'' PM 52T
Several other monitors are also available

* The 0.1× lens should be removed!

Comments on the equipment: The microscope setup suggested in **Table 3** may have to be adjusted individually for the different measurements that is planned. The board of the recommended microscope stand can be fastened to the microscope body in two different positions (**Figure 11**). This makes it possible to have a large selection of working distances between the table and the microscope objective, which is of great advantage when the capillaries of different regions of the body is going to be investigated.

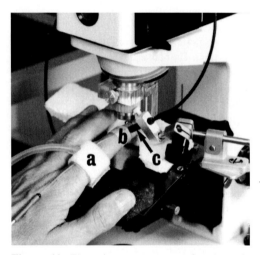

Figure 11. The microscope set up for dynamic capillaroscopy. The microscopy table can be tilted to a suitable angle. (a) Miniature cuff for arterial and venous occlusion. (b) Thermistor for measuring skin temperature. (c) Laser Doppler probe. See also **Figure 13**.

It is also recommended to build some kind of angled support that can be mounted on the microscope table. It should be constructed so that the proximal part of the investigated toe or finger is free for applying, say, a miniature blood pressure cuff or a thermistor onto the region.

A movable arm mounted on the microscope is recommended. With this arm other equipment, such as thermistors, laser Doppler probes, etc., can be applied close to the area observed by the microscope, for making simultaneous measurements (23).

Immobilization

When capillary blood cell velocity (CBV) is to be studied in human skin it is of great importance that the investigated object be as still as possible during the investigations. Immobilizing the part of the body that is studied is usually not enough, because there will always be some trembling in a living tissue, especially the hands and feet. In order to get the object still in relation to the microscope, it is therefore crucial to use some kind of firm connection between these two parts. The most successful support that has been describe so far is the so-called *finger holder* shown in **Figure 12** (and **Table 3**). It is composed of a plastic (or metal) holder and a firm, but flexible steel bracket (17, 63). The whole part can slide up and down the microscope objective and be fastened in the desired position by a screw. By using this gadget, it is possible to immobilize the area of observation almost completely with regard to the microscope system, facilitating the CBV measurements considerably. The bracket can be used successfully also in all other parts of the body investigated. As mentioned earlier, paraffin oil has to be applied to the area of observation in order to make the skin transparent

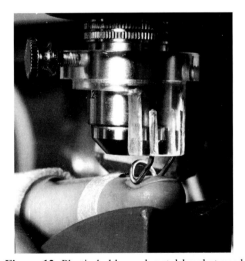

Figure 12. Plastic holder and metal bracket used to stabilize object under observation in the microscope. The holder can slide along the microscope objective and be stabilized in any suitable position.

Magnification

For optimal contrast and sharpness in the televised scene, a magnification of approximately 250× on a 5" monitor should be obtained. This magnification is also optimal for the computerized analysis system (CapiFlow®) described later in this section.

Recording System

The monitored field of view should be recorded on video tape for subsequent analysis. The video recorder should have the options of frame to frame, still picture, and search. The modern VHS system works nicely, although the U-matic system may have some advantages.

Examining Procedure

Investigation of Finger Nailfold Capillaries

The subject is examined in the supine or sitting position with the hand at heart level and after acclimation for 10–30 min in a room with a maintained temperature of 21–24°C. In most investigations, the third, fourth, or fifth finger of the left hand is used for examination because the skin of the fingers of the right hand are often traumatized, especially in people who work with their hands.

The arm and palm of the hand is placed on a soft, but firm, support on the investigation table. The fingers are positioned on the microscope table, and the finger chosen for investigation is placed under the microscope objective. Movements of the finger relative to the microscope are minimized by the use of the described bracket (**Figure 12**) that is attached to the microscope objective.

This bracket is crucial for getting a stable enough recording for making continuous measurements of blood cell velocity!

The nailfold capillaries are focused so that a clear picture can be seen on the TV monitor. Capillaries with good optical signals, i.e., with visible erythrocyte aggregates and plasma gaps, should be chosen for investigation. When suitable capillaries are seen on the TV monitor, the bracket on the objective is slid down to touch the finger nail and fixed in the suitable position. The microscope is then adjusted and the capillaries focused on the monitor screen.

Additional Equipment

If dynamic interventions are to be performed, some additional equipment must be applied to the examined finger. A 1.5–2 cm wide miniature cuff is applied around the base of the finger (**Figure 13**). The cuff should be connected to a reservoir ($\approx$ 2 l), a valve system, and a mercury blood pressure device in such a way that the occlusion pressure can be preset and the cuff instantly inflated or deflated. By this set up momentary arterial ($\approx$200 mmHg) or venous (50–60 mmHg) occlusions can be obtained at the base of the finger.

Temperature Measurements

The skin temperature of the area of observation should always be monitored. This can be done by a small thermistor that is fastened with a piece of tape as close to the area of observation as possible (**Figure 13**). We have used an electronic thermometer with digital display and an accuracy of 0.1°C (MC 8700, Exakon®, Copenhagen, Denmark). This instrument has two channels, which makes it possible to measure the room temperature and skin temperature simultaneously. When the thermistor is applied to the skin, it should be covered by some dark material (preferably a small piece of dark sponge) in order to avoid environmental influences on the recorded temperature.

Laser Doppler

During the past few years, the fiber optics of a laser Doppler (LD) apparatus (Periflux®, Perimed AB, Stockholm, Sweden) has also been applied close to the area of observation. The LD device records blood cell flux in the total microvascular bed of the skin. Most of the signal (90–95%) is generated by the movement of blood cells in the subpapillary vascular plexa (23). The combination of the LD fluxmetry and capillaroscopy makes it possible to study simultaneously dynamic fluctuations in the total skin

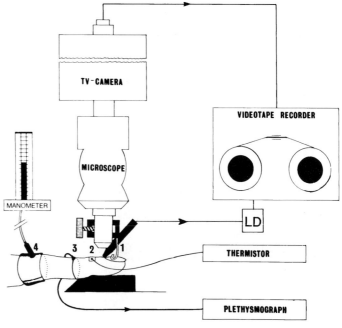

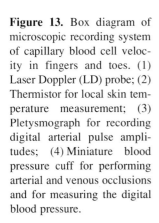

Figure 13. Box diagram of microscopic recording system of capillary blood cell velocity in fingers and toes. (1) Laser Doppler (LD) probe; (2) Thermistor for local skin temperature measurement; (3) Pletysmograph for recording digital arterial pulse amplitudes; (4) Miniature blood pressure cuff for performing arterial and venous occlusions and for measuring the digital blood pressure.

microcirculation and the nutritional capillaries of the same area (**Figure 13**).

Recording of Microscopic Images

When the investigation starts, the microscopic image that is produced on the monitor should be recorded on videotape for subsequent analysis. However, before the recording starts, it is recommended to check whether the signals in the capillary that is going to be used for measurements are good enough for analysis. This procedure is discussed in more detail below.

Data Processing

Capillary blood cell velocity (CBV) can be analyzed by several different techniques. A prerequisite for all these techniques is that there must be a good contrast difference between the moving objects in the capillary and the surrounding tissue. It is therefore crucial to obtain maximum contrast between moving red cells, white cells, and plasma gaps in the televised scene. Such an optimal picture is shown in **Figure 14**. In order to get an optimal contrast in the picture, the automatic adjustment of the TV camera has to be disconnected, and the light intensity and contrast manually adjusted to the best picture.

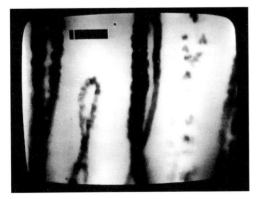

Figure 14. Photocopy of televised nailfold capillaries in a 76-year-old patient with cardiac insufficiency. Even single red cells can be seen.

Several different techniques have been used to record the movement of blood in the capillaries, and some of them are described here:

— mechanical devices,
— frame-to-frame analysis,
— flying spot technique,
— dual-window technique,
— cross-correlation method,
— computerized CBV measurements.

Mechanical Devices

The simplest technique for measuring the velocity is just to look at the passing particles and record, e.g., with a stopwatch, the time it takes for them to go from one point to another in the capillary. If the distance is known, the velocity can be calculated (40). This method can only be used at low and constant velocities, and these prerequisites are seldom present in living tissues.

The first time a mechanical device was used for measuring blood flow velocity in humans was in 1919 when Basler described a technique whereby a piece of hair was mechanically moved through the eyepiece of a microscope (1). The speed of the hair was synchronized with the speed of the blood cells and the velocity calculated. In 1934, Knisely (39), using a rotating cogwheel in the eyepiece instead of a hair, calculated the velocity of blood in animal preparations. However, because of their obvious limitations, these techniques have been seldom used in practice.

Frame-to-Frame Analysis

In this technique the videotape is moved in frame by frame, and the CBV is determined by measuring the displacement with time of plasma gaps, erythrocyte aggregates, or white cells in the capillary. In ordinary video recorders, the frame frequency is 50 per second, and the movement of a certain particle or gap along a defined distance can be calculated by measuring the number of frames that are needed for the signal to move along a predetermined distance.

The calculation is made according to the following formula (2, 7):

$$V = \frac{d}{t_2 - t_1}$$

where V = Velocity; d = distance; t_1 = time at start; t_2 = time after moving distance d.

Comments: As is easily understood the measurement with the frame to frame technique is extremely time consuming, and in practice only short sequences of CBV measurements can be performed. Because of this it is also practically impossible to record the spontaneous velocity fluctuations that arise, for example, from vasomotion in the precapillary vascular bed.

The Flying Spot Technique

The movement of blood corpuscles in the capillaries can also be measured by the so-called flying spot technique, which was first introduced by Brånemark and Jonsson in 1963 (5). They used an electronic scanner tube that projected the image of the flying spot into the path of the microscope. The spot could then be made to travel along the axis of the vessel under examination, and its speed was adjusted to coincide with the speed of the blood cells.

In 1982, Tyml and Ellis introduced the flying spot technique as a television method, whereby a special video marker equipment generates a train of small white windows on the television monitor (60). The windows can be regulated to move in any direction on the video screen and their speed manually adjusted on a continuous basis. The train of windows is position in parallel to a suitable capillary, the speed of the spots being synchronized with the speed of the moving blood cells or plasma gaps (**Figure 15**). The equipment is calibrated to the magnification on the TV monitor, after which the velocity can be calculated.

Comments: This technique can measure CBV in human skin capillaries from zero up to a maximum of about 1.3 mm/sec (34). As the CBV in human skin capillaries can vary from 0 to about 3 mm/sec, the technique has major limitations in clinical practice. Moreover, it is almost impossible to measure the normal fluctuations in CBV that are present in humans because of the vasomotion activity in the precapillary vascular beds. Therefore, only mean rest flow velocities can be calculated. As it is very easy to use the technique, it may, however, be convenient in some specific clinical situations (3, 35, 36).

The Dual-Window Technique

In this technique the video signal is past through a photometric analyzer that generates two photometric windows onto the TV monitor (**Figure 16**). The position of the windows can be manually adjusted both horizontally and vertically to a desired location along a suitable capillary, and can then be moved in tandem by means of an adjustable control, making it possible to correct for minor movements in the field of view (31, 32, 33). The interwindow distance can be modified, and it should be kept short for measuring low velocities and increased when higher velocities are calculated. For measuring CBV in human skin, the optimal distance between the windows is 10–50 µm (15, 63). The width of the windows should be modified to cover about 20% more than the diameter of the erythrocyte column in the capillary. For optimal

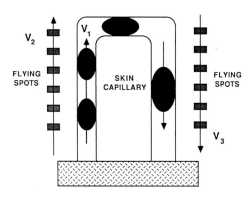

Figure 15. Schematic demonstration of the flying spot technique. The velocity of the flying spots (V2 and V3) is synchronized with the velocity of the blood cell aggregates (V1).

Dynamic Capillaroscopy Without Dyes

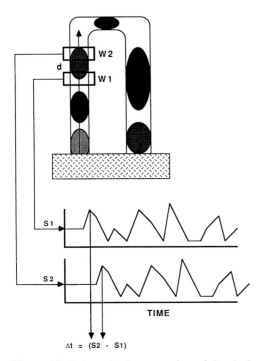

Figure 16. Schematic demonstration of the dual window technique for recording blood cell velocity in skin capillaries. S1 and S2 represent the signals generated by passing blood cells and plasma gaps in the upstream window (W1) and the downstream window (W2). The time delay (Δt) between S2 and S1 can be calculated into velocity if the distance (d) is known.

measuring conditions, the capillary limbs should be positioned vertically on the screen.

The video windows are sensitive to variations in the light intensity within the windows. Consequently, the passage of erythrocytes, leucocytes, and plasma gaps through the investigated capillary will give rise to variations in optical density, which are quantified by the windows and converted to electronic equivalents (**Figure 16**). The output from the windows can be recorded on a chart recorder. If the distance between the windows is known, the interwindow transit time, i.e., the time delay between similar events in the upstream and downstream windows, the velocity of blood cells or plasma gaps can be determined on a continuous basis. The formula for such calculations is:

$$\frac{a \times v_p}{b \times m} = CBV$$

where
a = the interwindow distance in mm on the TV monitor,
v_p = the paper speed,
b = the distance between identical events on the charts,
m = magnification on monitor.

Comments: If optimal contrast is present in the capillary, very distinct signals are registered on the chart recorder. If the speed of the paper is high (50–100 mm/sec), it is rather easy to measure the interwindow transit time manually, and the calculated velocity has a reasonable accuracy. The error of the velocity measurements with this method has been calculated with a rotating disc and found to be approximately 10% at a velocity of 0.5 mm/sec and a magnification of 250× on the monitor. The error is successively larger when the velocity increases. However, estimating CBV with this technique, as well as with the other two described, is very time consuming, though the CBV value obtained is rather exact. Measurements of CBV down to almost 0 mm/s is possible. Fast fluctuations in CBV can also be followed, because a value can usually be determined almost every second. To do this, however, it is better if the calculations are performed automatically, which can be done by the so-called cross-correlation technique.

Cross-Correlation Method

The technique of simplified cross-correlation was first described by Intaglietta and coworkers (31, 33), and in 1977 it was shown that it could be employed also for measuring CBV in human skin capillaries (17, 18, 19). The principle of the cross-correlation technique is the determination of the time interval by which the upstream signal has to be delayed to achieve maximum cross-correlation with the downstream signal (**Figure 16**). Different methods of correlation techniques have been used, one of which is described in the papers of Intaglietta and coworkers (31, 33). Through the cross-correlation technique, the velocity can be automatically calculated on a continuous basis for long periods. The principal of this and other techniques are nicely described in an article by Slaaf et al. in 1984 (59).

Accuracy of CBV measurements: The accuracy of CBV measurements has been tested by different methods. Bollinger et al. (2) estimated the accuracy of offline CBV measurements from videotapes by the frame-to-frame method to be within 15%. Butti et al. (7), comparing three different methods, including the cross-correlation technique, reported an experimental error on the order of 0.1 mm/sec. Östergren (63) found an excellent agreement (r=0.98) between the manual calculation of CBV by the dual window technique and mean CBV as read from the cross-correlator (IPM®, San Diego). However, it should be stressed that the commercially available cross-correlators have so far been very sophisticated, complicated, and difficult to use in clinical practice. One source of error lies in the interwindow distance, which must be carefully measured since 10% error in this measure produces a similar error in the obtained CBV values. Movements of the object relative to the microscope may also affect the accuracy of the measurements. Therefore, the use of the small bracket described on page 11 is crucial for obtaining good measurements.

Computerized CBV Measurements

So far, the equipment used for CBV measurements in humans has been based on standard photometric analyzers and velocity-tracking correlators. However, these systems need skilled operators to function, who are sometimes difficult to get when the measurements should be performed, e.g., in clinical practice.

During the past few years, a fully computerized system for doing these calculations has been developed (CapiFlow®, IM-CapiFlow, Stockholm). With this system, the whole process of CBV calculations is performed by the computer (24, 53). The dual-window technique is used for obtaining the signals, and the two photometric windows are generated by the computer program. The interwindow distance and the size of the windows can be modified, the distance between the windows being automatically given on the computer screen (**Figure 17**). The time delay is defined as the time corresponding to the peak value in the correlation function. CBV can be measured either as a function of time *(temporal correlation)* or as a function of distance *(spatial correlation)*. With both methods the CapiFlow® computes the velocity in real time every 20 ms, and presents updated values of the CBV graph 6.25 times every second. The correlation function is also

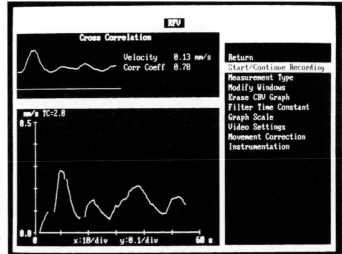

Figure 17. The computer menu for measuring CBV by the CapiFlow® system. The curve demonstrates an original CBV recording as it is generated by the computer.

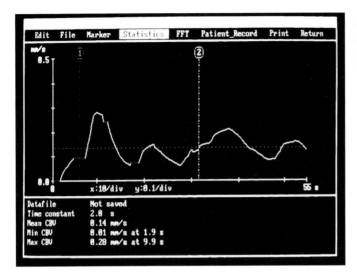

Figure 18. The computer screen showing a tracing of CBV from a nailfold capillary of a healthy subject.

```
CapiFlow   RFV

Name            :
Identity Code   :
Operator        :
Date            : January 11, 1990
Tape Nr/Pos     :
Comments        :
                :
```

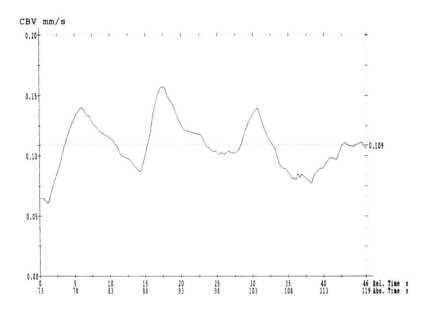

```
Datafile        : Not saved
Time Constant   :    2.0   s
Mean CBV        :    0.11  mm/s
Maximum CBV     :    0.16  mm/s
Minimum CBV     :    0.06  mm/s
```

Figure 19. Printer output showing a part of the CBV tracing from Figure 18.

displayed, this graph being redrawn every 1.28 s. Then the CBV values are given on the screen also with digits (**Figure 18**). If for some reason the windows are moved to another position, or the correlation function is too low to ensure adequate measurement quality, the velocity values are considered by the computer to be artefacts and displayed on the screen as a horizontal red line at the same velocity value as before the artefact appeared. This ensures that the given velocity values are correct; and when documented, all red lines are disregarded in the computerized mean velocity value given (**Figure 19**). The whole procedure of CBV measurement is controlled by the computer mouse or only a few keys on the computer keyboard. This makes the measurements extremely simple to handle even for persons with limited technical skills or computer knowledge.

Calculated Velocity Values

Resting Capillary Blood Cell Velocity (rCBV)

As mentioned earlier, rCBV in finger nailfold capillaries was calculated already in 1919 by Basler by a mechanical device (1), and the mean value he recorded was 0.60 mm/sec (range 0.11–1.2). Since then, several groups have measured the rCBV with all of the different techniques mentioned previously. The values achieved are presented in **Table 4**.

Comments: The mean values given in **Table 4** are similar for most studies. As can be seen, Richardsson (50) has a significantly lower value for CBV, but in this study there was an intentional selection of "low flow capillaries" resulting in the low values achieved. rCBV is highly dependent on two factors:

Table 4. Resting capillary blood cell velocity (rCBV) in human finger nailfold as evaluated by several different techniques.

Investigator	Year	rCBV mm/s (range)	n	Method
Basler	1919	0.6 (art.) (0.11–1.2)	5	mechanical
Bollinger et al.	1974	0.84 (art.) (0.39–1.74) 0.47 (ven.) (0.24–0.83)	5	frame to frame
Butti et al.	1975	0.8 (0.14–2.36)	5	frame to frame cross-correlation
Fagrell et al.	1977	0.65 (0.12–2.6)	12	cross-correlation
Richardson	1982	0.2*	30	,, ,,
Jacobs	1985	0.66 (0.21–0.98)**	25	flying spot
Mahler et al.	1986	0.66 (0.05–1.1)**	25	flying spot
Östergren & Fagrell	1986	0.67 (men) 0.53 (women) (0.01-2.8)	33 31	cross-correlation

* In this study capillaries with low velocity were chosen in order to get the best signals.
** The flying spot technique cannot measure values >1.3 mm/s.

— Diameter of the Capillary

As the diameter of skin capillaries varies from ≈7–≈ 20 μm in the nailfolds, this influences rCBV considerably. Every individual capillary also varies in diameter from the arterial to venous end. Bollinger et al. (2, 7) recorded an average rCBV of 0.84 mm/s in the arterial limb (Ø = 12 μm) and 0.47 mm/sec in the venous part (Ø = 15 μm) of nailfold capillaries. Fagrell et al. (17, 18) recorded a mean CBV of 0.65 mm/sec in the arterial limb close to the apex of the capillary. The mean skin temperature in the area under observation in this study was 30.4°C. In the study by Bollinger et al., the skin temperature was not measured. **Figure 20** shows how the velocity decreases along seven capillaries from the arterial to the venous end. As can be seen, rCBV in the distal venous limb is only about 25% of the value in the proximal arterial limb.

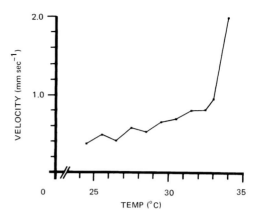

Figure 21. Demonstration of the successive increase in capillary blood cell velocity with temperature in a single nailfold capillary of a healthy subject. Notice the marked increase of velocity occuring at 34°C. (Reprinted by permission from 15.)

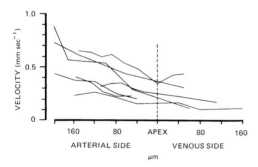

Figure 20. Capillary blood cell velocity along seven nailfold capillaries of healthy subjects. The velocity decreases successively from the arterial to the venous limb of the capillary because of an increase in vessel diameter. (Reprinted by permission from 15.)

— Temperature of the Skin

The local skin temperature also influences rCBV substantially. As can be seen in **Figure 21**, rCBV increases successively up to a skin temperature of about 30–32°C after which temperature there is a dramatic velocity increase (15, 17, 63). Consequently, when rCBV is used, the temperature of the investigated area has to be recorded.

Furthermore, our findings indicate that rCBV varies as a function of time because of the vasomotion activity in the precapillary vascular beds. The result of this activity is shown in the rCBV values as variations in flow velocity. The only method that can continuously record these variations in rCBV is the automatic cross-correlation technique. The measurement of rCBV has been still more simplified by the use of the CapiFlow® computer system. When a recording of rCBV has been performed over the investigation period, the computer automatically evaluates mean, minimum, and maximum velocity, and displays them on the TV screen (**Figure 18**), and a graph can also be printed out (**Figure 19**).

— Pulse Components of Capillary Blood Cell Velocity

In most literature on basic physiology, it is stated that the arterial pulse wave is damped out before it reaches the nutritional capillaries. However, this is not the case in the capillaries of the skin, where the influence of the arterial pulse is prominent both in finger nailfold capillaries and in the capillaries of the lower leg (17, 19). At higher skin temperatures, the influence of the arterial pulse wave on rCBV is often

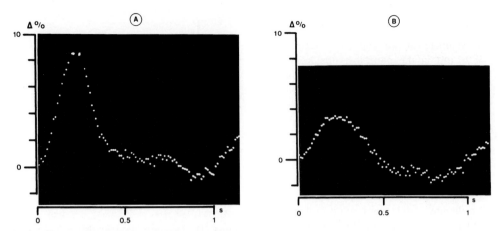

Figure 22. Influence of arterial pulses on CBV in a nailfold capillary of a healthy subject. The figure shows the averaged pulsatile flow components during 128 cardiac cycles. In (A) the skin temperature was 32.8°C, and CBV is markedly influenced by the digital pulse. In (B) the temperature was only 24.8°C, and the influence of the arterial pulse is significantly reduced.

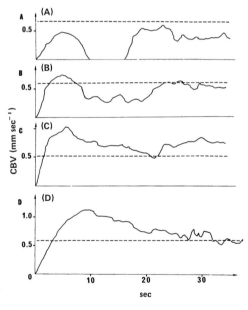

Figure 23. Postocclusive reactive hyperemia response after 15 s (A), 30 s (B), 60 s (C), and 120 s (D). At short occlusions (A and B), no repayment of flow is seen, and after about 10–15 s flow sometimes (A) stops completely for 5–10 s. At longer occlusions (C–D), a reactive hyperemia response can be seen and the vasoconstricting phase is abandoned (21).

marked, while at lower temperatures the precapillary vascular bed is more constricted and the effect of the pulse wave on rCBV weaker (**Figure 22**).

— **Flow Motion Activity**

Rhythmic variations in the skin microcirculation have been observed and are described further on page 25.

Postocclusive Reactive Hyperaemia (PRH)

An arterial occlusion of the digital arteries can be performed in a digit by means of a miniature cuff (2 cm wide) placed around the base of the finger or the toe. Various occlusion durations from 15 s up to 6 min have been performed (21). As shown in **Figure 23**, at short occlusions CBV during reactive hyperemia do not regularly exceed the resting CBV before occlusion. In about 80% of normal subjects, the flow also stops completely 10–25 s after cuff release. This reaction is most probably caused by a sudden increase in transmural pressure when cuff pressure is released, resulting in a stretching of the vascular smooth muscle cells and leading to a reflex vasoconstriction, called the myogenic response during RH (38, 63, 64). After longer occlusions, metabolic factors become more involved and seem to counteract the myogenic response. Quite another pattern can be seen (**Figure 23**) with a successive increase of the peak and the duration of CBV during the PRH. A number of different substances, such as potassium, adenosine, histamine, substance P, and prostaglandins, have been suggested as a mediator of this reaction. Several of these factors, together with the reduced oxygen tension in itself, most probably contribute to the response.

The responses to still longer occlusions have been studied by Romanus (52) in human skin tubes by intravital microscopy. Circulatory arrests were produced in the skin tubes for 1–6 h. When cuff pressure was released after 1 and 2 h of ischemia, the circulation started within a few seconds, and a hyperemic reaction could be seen for almost 30 min. Even after 6 h of ischemia blood flow started, though the velocities varied considerably and no clear hyperemic reaction could be seen. These results indicate that the skin tissue is extremely resistant to ischemia, which was pointed out already in 1961 by Burton (6) who stated that "an actual cessation of all blood flow must be present before skin necrosis occurs."

— **One-Minute Arterial Occlusion**

For the study of the PRH in finger or toe nailfold capillaries, a one-minute arterial occlusion has been found in clinical studies to be optimal (15, 17–23, 63, 64). This occlusion time mostly involves the myogenic reaction to ischemia and in normal subjects gives a clear-cut peak because of a moderate secondary vasoconstriction. The time to the peak is very constant (7.8 ± 2.4 s) in healthy subjects. However, the percent increase of CBV above the resting value varies and is highly dependent on the local skin temperature. At higher temperatures (>30°C), where the resting CBV is already elevated because of a local vasodilatation, the PRH response is limited—and at about 34°C the response is almost completely gone (**Figure 24**). The normal PRH response has been found to be disturbed significantly in several pathologically conditions (further discussed in Part 2).

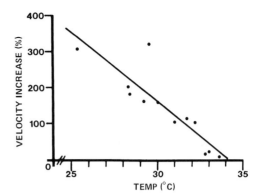

Figure 24. Correlation between skin temperature and peak velocity (% above resting value) during postocclusive reactive hyperemia after a 1 min arterial occlusion. At higher temperratures, there is almost no reactive hyperemia response at all. (Reprinted by permission from 15.)

The parameters found to be the most useful in human studies are shown in **Figure 25a** and **Table 5**.

Venous Occlusion

Occlusion of the venous outflow of blood from the investigated region can be performed by inflating the miniature cuff at the base of the digit to 50 or 60 mmHg (63, 64). This procedure triggers the so-called veno-arteriolar reflex, through which a constriction of the precapillary arterioles is induced by the sudden increase in local venous pressure (22, 25). The occlusion duration most often used is 30 s, during which time the CBV is continuously recorded (**Figure 25b**). The results are expressed as a percentage of the mean rCBV before the occlusion. The normal reaction is that CBV falls when occlusion reaches a nadir in 3.5–8.5 s, where flow stops for a few seconds in about 70% of normals. During the rest of the occlusion period, flow slowly increases, and mean CBV during the whole 30-s period is usually about 25% of preocclusion CBV (**Table 5**). This reaction has also been found to be pathologically disturbed, for example, in diabetics.

Figure 25. (a) Schematic drawing of the different parameters used in clinical dynamic capillaroscopy. For explanation of abbreviations, see **Table 5**.

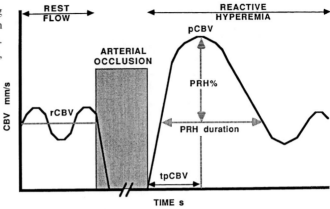

(b) Schematic drawing of CBV reaction during 30 s of venous occlusion.

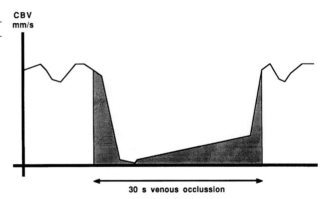

Table 5. Suitable parameters for measuring the reactivity of blood flow in human nutritional skin capillaries. See also Figure 25A.

Abbreviation	Explanation	Normal values
rCBV (mm/s)	CBV during rest	see Table 4
pCBV (mm/s)	Peak CBV after a 1 min arterial occlusion at the base of the finger or toe	Depends on temperature See page 20
tpCBV (s)	Time to pCBV during PRH	7.8 ± 2.4
PRH (%)	The percent increase of CBV above rCBV during PRH	Depends on temperature See page 21
PRH duration	The time CBV is higher than rCBV during PRH	Depends on the occlusion duration
VO% (%)	Mean CBV during venous occlusion	24 ± 6

Cooling Procedures

Contralateral Cooling

This test is used for studying the reflex mechanism of cooling (22, 64). A finger of the left hand is investigated under the microscope. After a steady period of 10–15 min baseline values should be recorded. The contralateral hand is then immersed in water at 5–15°C for 1–5 min. The time of immersion can be varied, and generally it is the initial phase of the cooling procedure that is interesting for evaluating the reflex mechanism. After withdrawal of the hand, the CBV should be continuously recorded for another 3–5 min.

— **Cooling at 15°C**

The baseline CBV has been measured in seven healthy nonsmoking volunteers, aged 21–41 years (22). Before cooling, rCBV was 0.52 ± 0.22 mm/s. The skin temperature was 30.3°C. When the contralateral hand was immersed in water of 15°C, CBV decreased to 0.37 ± 0.15 mm/s (n.s.). The CBV immediately became more irregular, and in three subjects blood cell standstill was observed for short periods (3–7 s). The skin temperature in the investigated finger fell slightly to 29.5°C and continued to fall after withdrawal of the hand to 28.9°C (n.s.).

— **Cooling at 4°C**

Before contralateral cooling in 4°C the rCBV was 0.30 ± 0.07 mm/s and the skin temperature 28.9°C (22). CBV decreased during the cooling procedure to 0.20 ± 0.05 mm/s ($p<0.001$). Blood cell standstill was now observed in all subjects for 2–30 s, with a frequency of 2–6 times/min. After cooling, CBV remained low (0.26 ± 0.06 mm/s) while the skin temperature was unchanged.

Comments: The test of cooling the contralateral hand may be used for studying disturbances of the skin microvascular reactivity in several diseased states. It is easy to perform and to reproduce, though it can cause some discomfort to subjects when low temperatures are used.

Direct Cooling

— **Cold Water**

CBV has also been studied after direct cooling of the finger. The hand and fingers were immersed in cold water, and immediately after this provocation CBV was determined every 15 s until the velocity reached the preprovocation value. Jacobs (34) used this technique to study differences between healthy subjects and patients with Raynaud's phenomenon.

— **Cold Air**

A more sophisticated technique to evaluate the effect of cold on CBV is described by Mahler et al. (43). CO_2 is used as a cooling medium. By rapid decompression of liquid CO_2 during the outflow from a pressure tank, the gas drops in temperature in a predictive way. The tank pressure should exceed 6 ATN, and the gas flow rate should be 50 l/min. With this prerequisite –10°C will be reached in the gas outflow after 2 min. Cooling is then continued for 60 s, after which the temperature has dropped to –20°C.

Before cooling, the hand is immersed in a water bath of 40°C for 3 min to standardize the local temperature conditions. The hand should be covered by a plastic glove. rCBV is measured continuously for 3 min before cooling, and then recorded during the whole cooling procedure where standstill periods and CBV are calculated. After cooling, rCBV is continuously calculated for another 2–3 min. The periods of flow stop and CBV have been found to be very reproducible (r=0.89). The values recorded by Mahler et al. (43) are given in **Table 6**.

Table 6. CBV values in healthy control subjects during local cooling test according to Mahler et al. (43) (n=25).

	Normal values
rCBV before cooling	0.66 ± 0.25 mm/s
CBV during cooling	0.15 ± 0.06 mm/s
Stop frequency	1/25
Stop duration	1.9 s

Chapter 1.2

Comments: The technique has been used for studying the disturbances of skin microvascular reactivity in different types of Raynaud's syndrome. The sensitivity and specificity of the test has been found to be 0.95, and it also appears to be very sensitive for evaluating the effect of therapeutic interventions (3, 43). Differences between primary and secondary Raynaud's phenomenon can also be clearly documented by the technique (43).

Evaluation of Relative Hematocrit in Human Capillaries

Methods were developed during the 1970s for studying hematocrit variations in the microcirculation of experimental animals (37). Such studies revealed a marked variation in the hematocrit of single capillaries, and it was found that the hematocrit in mesenteric capillaries of cat changed almost constantly and was closely related to the CBV in the capillaries.

Fagrell et al. (20, 23) used the described dual-window, video-densitometric technique for simultaneous evaluation of CBV and hematocrit in human skin capillaries.

Investigation Procedure

CBV measurements are performed with the cross-correlation technique from the videotapes; a schematic presentation of the technique is given in **Figure 26**. The hematocrit (Hct) for each capillary is deduced from continuous records of the video-densitometric output of one (A1) of the video windows. A third video window (B) is positioned over an area adjacent to the capillary. The purpose of this window is to record any fluctuations in the optical density of the tissue surrounding the capillaries. These may be caused by variations in the light intensity or the focusing of the monitored scene.

Zero hematocrit is established by recording the output of the window positioned over the capillary (A1) in the absence of erythrocytes. In order to provide meaningful information on the mean hematocrit variation over a certain period,

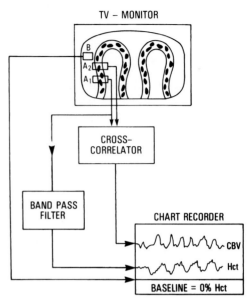

Figure 26. Box diagram showing the principal of combined CBV and relative hematocrit (Hct) measurements in single nailfold capillaires (20).

the signal from individual red cells or cell aggregates must be filtered away. This is achieved by passing the signal from the video window through a low-pass filter with an upper limit of 0.6 Hz. By this procedure, only the DC shift in the window (i.e., the mean density of red cells) is recorded (**Figure 26**). In human skin capillaries it is possible for more than one cell to pass the video windows at the same time. Consequently, some erythrocytes may be in the shadow of others and are not seen by the video window. This makes it impossible to record the absolute volume hematocrit in the capillary. The relative highest density can be determined for each single capillary. This value, which is the minimum (= darkest) output from the window recorded during the registration period, is called the 100% relative hematocrit for the capillary.

Hematocrit Variations

In most skin capillaries of humans, the hematocrit varies almost constantly. The variations seem to be most pronounced in capillaries with

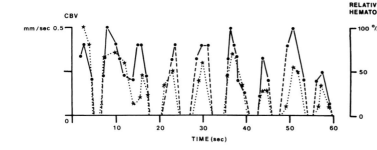

Figure 27. Simultaneous recording of CBV and relative hematocrit in a single human nailfold capillary. Notice the strong correlation between CBV and relative hematocrit variations (20).

a small diameter. In about half of the capillaries the hematocrit and CBV vary periodically with a frequency of about 6–10 c/min. These fluctuations are sometimes so strong that the flow becomes intermittent (**Figure 27**).

Hematocrit and CBV

A close relationship has been noticed between Hct and CBV (**Figure 28**). When CBV increases, Hct increases and vice versa. The two variables are, however, shifted in phase to a greater or smaller degree. This is mainly because of the position of the window on the capillary: When it is placed over the most proximal part of the capillary, the phase shift is less marked than when it is positioned over the distal, venous part. The reason for this is that when the window is closer to the region where the activity of vasomotion is located, i.e., the precapillary arterioles, the time for the blood cells to reach the recording window is shorter.

Comments: It has been shown that the relative hematocrit in most human capillaries varies to a great extent from one moment to another. Similar observations have been seen also in the microcirculation of animal preparations (37). The high correlation between CBV and Hct results most probably because both these variables are primarily regulated by the same mechanism—the vasomotor tone in the precapillary arterioles and metarterioles.

From the results achieved, it is found that each capillary seems to have an individual vasomotion activity. Capillaries within the same televised scene are likely to be fed from the same incoming arteriole. Nevertheless, Hct and CBV can vary substantially from one capillary to another (**Figure 28**). This is a further indication that the vasomotion activity seen is most probably produced by activity at the precapillary arteriolar level.

Flow Motion Activity

During the past decade, great interest have been devoted to the rhythmic oscillations of flow in the human skin (23, 58). However, most of the information concerning flow motion in humans has been studied not by capillaroscopy, but by other techniques. Fagrell et al. studied the flow motion activity using laser Doppler (LD) fluxmetry and dynamic capillary microscopy (23). The relationship between events seen in the LD and capillary blood cell velocity (CBV) curves were analyzed from the skin of fingers of 14 healthy subjects. By using computerized frequency analysis, the relationship between the two sets of data could be calculated. The results showed that there was a linear relationship between the two techniques ($p<0.05$–0.001) in 11 out 14 sets of records. The importance of the vasomotion activity in clinical practice is thus far not fully understood, though significant differences in the vasomotion pattern have been observed in healthy subjects and patients with, for example, peripheral arterial insufficiency (58). The flow motion pattern has been studied also in newborn infants by dynamic capillary microscopy (49). It was found that the CBV is much more steady in newborns and does not have the normal vasomotion pattern seen in adult subjects. The reason for this may be that the microvascular bed of the skin is not fully developed in the newborn infant. Further stud-

Figure 28. Simultaneous recording of CBV and relative hematocrit (Hct) in three different capillaries in the same field of view. Notice that the pattern differ between capillaries 1 and 3 in the middle part of the tracing. (Reprinted by permission from 15.)

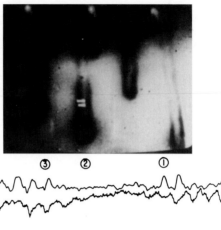
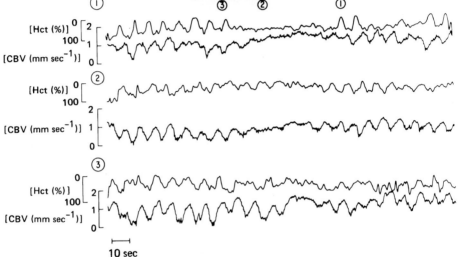

ies of flow motion in the skin microcirculation must be performed in order to evaluate the importance of this parameter in clinical practice.

The Effect of Smoking on CBV

The CBV has been studied in regular smokers (more than 5 cigarettes/day) and nonsmokers (63). The smokers had refrained from smoking for at least 2 h proceeding the investigation. It was found that the CBV during rest or post-occlusive reactive hyperemia was no different in the two groups, which is in agreement with the finding that tobacco smoking reduces the total skin blood flow acutely, but that the effect is not longlasting (51). As the subjects had refrained from smoking for 2 h prior to the investigation, no effects on microvascular hemodynamics were to be expected.

The acute effect of smoke inhalation on CBV in human skin has been studied by Richardsson (51). He studied capillary blood flow (capillary cross sectional area × flow velocity) and found that all kind of cigarettes significantly reduced capillary blood flow with a maximal effect within the first 2 min of the postsmoking period ($p<0.05$). There was no significant difference between low-, medium-, and high-nicotine cigarettes, and it was concluded that the effect on capillary blood flow is not related to the nicotine content of the cigarettes. The effect on capillary blood flow also seems to be much less than the effect on total digital blood flow.

CBV in Full-Term Neonates

Very little is known about microcirculation in infancy. It has been reported that in neonates peripheral blood flow is high, but blood pressure low, which is rather confusing (41). The blood rheology is also unique in neonates, the peripheral hematocrit being higher than the central one (41). It is therefore of great clinical interest to study the circulation in the nutritional capillaries of neonates. This has been made possible by capillaroscopy. Simultaneous recordings of CBV, skin temperature, blood pressure, and hematocrit has been performed to determine when the normal variations in these parameters affect the CBV. Norman et al. (49) investigated 43 full-term infants of normal weight, all with a history of uncomplicated vaginal deliveries after normal pregnancies. The study period was 2–7 days of postnatal age.

The mean CBV for all infants was 0.38 ± 0.21 mm/s with a range from 0.004–1.2 mm/s in individual capillaries. No sex difference was found, but the CBV was somewhat (n.s.) faster for boys (0.42 mm/s) than for girls (0.34 mm/s). The hematocrit in the skin was 60 ± 7% and ranged from 43–80%. There was a decrease from 64% on day 2 to 54% on day 7 (p<0.01), and CBV increased successively during this period. According to multiple regression analyses, this could be attributed to the age-related drop in hematocrit. A significantly lower CBV was observed in the neonates with an increased hematocrit (p<0.001), but the relationship was nonlinear (**Figure 29**). In the child with the highest hematocrit (80%), the CBV was very slow, and the capillary flow stopped completely at intervals of up to a duration of 40 s. Similar results have also been noticed in adult subjects with very high hematocrit (see page 144).

Comments: Studies of the skin capillaries in neonates have indicated poor skin capillary vascularization (49). Despite this, rapid changes have been demonstrated in the neonatal limb and total skin blood flows after temperature alterations, indicating a mature vascular response (49). Such alterations in CBV could not be found, and there was no relationship to skin temperature. Thus, the higher total peripheral blood flow seen in newborn infants is more likely to bypass superficial skin capillaries through deeper vascular beds, which suggests an increased flow resistance in neonatal skin capillaries. These findings suggest that the thermoregulation under normal conditions is not mediated via blood flow changes in the superficial skin capillaries, so that deductions of the normal skin capillary perfusion cannot be made from skin temperature measurements.

References 1.1 and 1.2

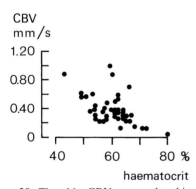

Figure 29. The skin CBV versus the skin-prick hematocrit in neonates. A significant correlation was found between the two parameters (r=–0.50, p<0.001), and after log-transformation of the CBV (r=–0.64, p<0.001) (Reprinted with permission from Norman et al., 49.)

1) Basler, A.: Über die Bestimmung der Strömungsgeschwindigkeit in den Blutkapillallen der menschlichen Haut. *Muench. Med. Wochenschr.* 13, 347–348, 1919.

2) Bollinger, A., Butti, P., Barras, J. P., Trachsler, H., Siegenthaler, W.: Red blood cell velocity in nailfold capillaries of man measured by a television microscopy technique. *Microvasc. Res.* 7, 61–72, 1974.

3) Boss, C., Schneuwly, P., Mahler, F.: Evaluation and clinical application of the flying spot method in clinical nailfold capillary TV microscopy. *Int. J. Microcirc.: Clin. Exp.* 6, 15–24, 1987.

4) Brånemark, P. I.: The contribution of microscopes to the study of living circulation: Contributions and limitations of refined classical methods. *J. Royal Microscopic. Soc.* 83, 29–35, 1964.

5) Brånemark, P. I., Jonsson, I.: Determination of the velocity of corpuscles in blood capillaries. *Biorheology* 1, 143–146, 1963.
6) Burton, A. C.: Special features of the circulation of the skin. In: Montagna W. & Ellis R. A. (eds.): *Blood vessels and circulation. Vol. II. Advances in biology of the skin.* Pergamon Press, New York, 117–122, 1961.
7) Butti P., Intaglietta M., Reimann H., Holliger C. H., Bollinger A., Anliker M.: Capillary red blood cell velocity measurements in human nailfold by video densitometric method. *Microvasc. Res.* 10, 1–8, 1975.
8) Conrad, M. C.: Abnormalities of the digital vasculature as related to ulceration and gangrene. *Circulation* 88, 568–581, 1968.
9) Conrad, M. C.: *Functional anatomy of the circulation to the lower extremities.* Year Book Medical Publishers Inc., Chicago, 1971.
10) Davis, M. J., Lawler, J. C.: The capillary circulation of the skin. *Arch. Dermatol.* 77, 690–703, 1958.
11) Davis, E., Landau, J.: *Clinical capillary microscopy.* Charles C. Thomas, Springfield, IL, 1966
12) Fagrell, B.: Vital capillaroscopy—A clinical method for studying changes of skin microcirculation in patients suffering from vascular disorders of the leg. *Angiology* 23, 284–298, 1972.
13) Fagrell, B.: Vital capillary microscopy—A clinical method for studying changes of the nutritional skin capillaries in legs with arteriosclerosis obliterans. *Scand. J. Clin. Lab. Invest. Suppl.* 133, 1973.
14) Fagrell, B.: Local microcirculation in chronic venous incompetence and leg ulcers. *Vasc. Surg.* 13, 217–225, 1979.
15) Fagrell, B.: Microcirculation of the skin. Chapter VI in Mortillaro, A. N. (ed.): *The physiology and pharmacology of the microcirculation.* Academic Press, Orlando, FL, 1984.
16) Fagrell, B., Lund, F.: Vital capillary microscopy as a test method for therapeutic procedures in peripheral vascular diseases. In *Clinical evaluation of testing methods of vasoactive drugs effects.* C.E.P.I., Rome, pp. 329–334, 1968.
17) Fagrell, B., Fronek, A., Intaglietta, M.: A microscope television system for studying flow velocity in human skin capillaries. *Am. J. Physiol.* 233, H318–H321, 1977.
18) Fagrell, B., Fronek, A., Intaglietta, M.: Capillary blood flow velocity during rest and post-occlusive reactive hyperemia in skin areas of the toes and lower. *Bibl. Anat.* 16, 159–161, 1977.
19) Fagrell, B., Fronek, A., Intaglietta, M.: Capillary flow components and reactive hyperemia studied by clinical microscopy. *Bibl. Anat.* 16, 112–115, 1977.
20) Fagrell, B., Intaglietta, M., Östergren, J.: Relative hematocrit in human skin capillaries and its relation to capillary blood flow velocity. *Microvasc. Res.* 20, 327–335, 1980.
21) Fagrell, B., Östergren, J.: Reactive hyperemia response in human skin capillaries after varying occlusion duration. *Bibl. Anat.* 20, 692–696, 1981.
22) Fagrell, B., Svedman, P., Östergren, J.: The influence of hydrostatic pressure and contralateral cooling on capillary blood cell velocity and transcutaneous oxygen tension in fingers. *Int. J. Microcirc.: Clin. Exp.* 1, 163–171, 1982.
23) Fagrell, B., Intaglietta, M, Tsai, A. G., and Östergren, J.: Combination of laser Doppler flowmetry and capillary microscopy for evaluating the dynamics of skin microcirculation. *Prog. Appl. Microcirc.* No. 11: 125–138 (Karger, Basel) 1986.
24) Fagrell, B., Eriksson, S.E., Malmström, S., Sjölund, A.: Computerized data analysis of capillary blood cell velocity. *Int. J. Microcirc.: Clin. Exp.* 7, 276, 1988.
25) Gaskell, P., Burton, A. C.: Local postural vasomotor reflexes arising from the limb veins. *Circulat. Res.* 1, 27–39, 1953.
26) Gilje, O.: Ulcus cruris in venous circulatory disturbances. *Acta. Derm. Venereol. Suppl.* 22, 1–328, 1949.
27) Gilje, O.: Capillaroscopy in the differential diagnosis of skin diseases. *Acta. Derm. Venereol.* 33, 303–317, 1953.
28) Heuter, C.: Die Cheilo Angioskopie, eine neue Untersuchungsmethode zu physiolo-

gischen. *ZBL. Med. Wiss.* 17, 225–230, 1879.
29) Heisig, N.: Untersuchungen über das mikrovaskuläre System bei degenerativen Gefäßkrankungen. *Arch Kreisl.-Forsch* 47, 95–137, 1965.
30) Houtman, P. M.: *Microvascular and immunological studies in Raynaud's phenomenon.* Thesis, Rijksuniversiteit Groningen. Drukkerij van Denderen B.V., Groningen, The Netherlands, 1985.
31) Intaglietta, M., Tompkins, W. R., Richardson, D. R.: Velocity measurements in the microvasculature of the cat omentum by on-line method. *Microvasc. Res.* 2, 462–473, 1970.
32) Intaglietta, M., Tompkins, W. R.: Microvascular measurements by video image shearing and splitting. *Microvasc. Res.* 5, 309–312, 1973.
33) Intaglietta, M., Silverman, N. R., Tompkins, W. R.: Capillary flow velocity measurements in vivo and in situ by television methods. *Microvasc. Res.* 10, 165–179, 1975.
34) Jacobs, M.: *Capillary microscopy and hemorheology in vasospastic and occlusive vascular diseases.* Thesis, St. Annadal Hospital, Limburg University, Maastricht, The Netherlands, 1985.
35) Jacobs, M., Slaaf, D., Lemmens, J., Reneman, R.: The use of hemorheological and microcirculatory parameters in evaluating the effect of treatment in Raynaud's phenomenon. *Vasc. Surg.* 21, 9–15, 1987
36) Jacobs, M., Jörning, P., Joshi, S., Kitslaar, P., Slaaf, D., Reneman, R.: Epidural spinal cord electrical stimulation improves microvascular blood flow in severe limb ischemia. *Ann. Surg.* 207, 179–183, 1988.
37) Johnson, P. C., Blaschke, J., Burton, K. S., Dial, J. H.: Influence of flow variations on capillary hematocrit in mesentery. *Am. J. Physiol.* 221, 105–112, 1971.
38) Johnson, P. C., Burton, K. S., Henrich, H.: Effect of occlusion duration on reactive hyperemia in sartorius muscle capillaries. *Am. J. Physiol.* 230(3), 715–719, 1976.
39) Knisely, M. H., Barnes, R. H., Satterwhite, Jr., W. M.: In vivo observations of the bulbar conjunctival blood vessels and blood of functioning people 60 years of age and over. *J. Geront.* 12, 429–436, 1957.
40) Lee, R. E., Holtze, E. A.: Peripheral vascular system in bulbar conjunctiva of young normotensive adults at rest. *J. Clin. Invest.* 29, 146–150, 1950.
41) Linderkamp, O., Versmold, H., Riegel, K., Betke, K.: Contributions of red cell and plasma to blood viscosity in preterm and full-term infants and adults. *Pediatrics* 74, 45–50, 1984.
42) Lombard, W. P.: The blood pressure in the arterioles, capillaries, and small veins of the human skin. *Am. J. Physiol.* 29, 335–362, 1912.
43) Mahler, F., Sanner, H., Annaheim, M., Linder, H. R.: Capilloroscopic evaluation of erythrocyte flow velocity in patients with Raynaud's syndrome by means of a local cold exposure test. *Prog. appl. Microcirc.* 11, 47–59, 1986.
44) Mahler, F., Nagel, G., Saner, H., Kneubühl, F.: In vivo comparison of the nailfold capillary diameters as determined by using the erythrocyte column and FITC-labelled albumin. *Int. J. Microcirc.: Clin. Exp.* 2, 147–155, 1983.
45) Maricq, HR.: Widefield capillary microscopy. Technique and rating scale for abnormalities seen in scleroderma and related disorders. *Arthritis. Rheum.* 24, 1159–1165, 1981.
46) Maricq, H. R. Nailfold capillary photography. *Prog. appl. Microcirc.* 11, 11–27, 1986.
47) McCulloch, J. C., Pashby, T. J.: The significance of conjunctival aneurysm in diabetes. *Brit. J. Ophthal.* 34, 495, 1950.
48) Müller, O.: *Die feinstein Blutgefässe des Menschen in gesunden und kranken Tagen.* F. Enke Verlag, Stuttgart, Vol. 1,2, 1937/1939.
49) Norman, M., Herin, P., Fagrell, B., Zetterström, R.: Skin capillary blood cell velocity in full-term infants its relation to skin temperature, blood pressure, hematocrit and postnatal age. *Pediat. Res.* 23, 585–588, 1988.
50) Richardson, D.: Relationship between digital artery and nailfold capillary flow veloci-

ties in human skin. *Microcirculation* 2, 283–296, 1982.
51) Richardson, D.: Effects of tobacco smoke inhalation on capillary blood flow in human skin. *Archs envir. Hlth.* 42,19–27, 1987.
52) Romanus, M.: *Microcirculatory reactions to local pressure induced ischemia. A vital microscopic study in hamster cheek pouch and a pilot study in man.* Thesis. Acta Chir. Scand. Suppl. 479, 1977.
53) Rosén, L., Fagrell, B., Eriksson, S., Sjölund, A.: Evaluation of a completely computerized cross-correlation technique for measuring capillary blood cell velocity in humans. *Int. J. Microcirc.: Clin Exp.*, in press.
54) Rothman, S.: Chapter 4 in *Physiology and biochemistry of the skin.* Univ. of Chicago Press, Chicago, 1954.
55) Ryan, T. J.: The epidermis and its blood supply in venous disorders of the leg. *Trans. St. John's Hosp. Derm. Soc.* (London) 55, 51, 1969.
56) Ryan, T. J., Copeman, P. W. M.: Microvascular pattern and blood stasis in skin disease. *Brit. J. Derm.* 81, 563, 1969.
57) Ryan, T. J., Kurban, A. K.: New vessel growth in the adult skin. *Brit. J. Derm.* 82, 92–98, 1970.
58) Seifert, H., Jäger, K., Bollinger, A.: Analysis of flow motion by the laser Doppler technique in patients with peripheral arterial occlusion disease. *Int. J. Microcirc.: Clin Exp.* 7, 223–236, 1988.
59) Slaaf, D. W., Arts, T., Jeurens, T. J. M., Tangelder, G. J., Reneman, R. S.: Electronic measurement of red blood cell velocity and volume flow in microvessels. In Chayen J. & Bitensky L. (eds.): *Investigative microtechniques in medicine and biology. Vol 1.* Marcel Dekker, New York, 1984.
60) Tyml, K., Ellis, C. G.: Evaluation of the flying spot technique as a television method for measuring red cell velocity in microvessels. *Int. J. Microcirc.: Clin. Exp.* 1, 145–155, 1982.
61) Weiss, E., Müller, O.: Über Beobachtung der Hautkapillaren und ihre klinische Bedeutung. *Münch. Med. Wshr.* 1, 609, 1917
62) Zimmer, J. G., Demis, D. J.: The study of the physiology and pharmacology of the human cutaneous microcirculation by capillary microscopy and television cinematography. *Angiology* 15, 232–235, 1964.
63) Östergren, J.: *Studies on skin capillary blood cell velocity by video photometric capillaroscopy.* Thesis, Repro Print, Stockholm, Sweden, 1984.
64) Östergren, J., Fagrell, B., Svedman, P.: The influence of venous and arterial occlusion on skin capillary blood flow on transcutaneous oxygen tension in fingers. *Int. J. Microcirc.: Clin. Exp.* 2, 315–324, 1983.

1.3 Dynamic Capillaroscopy with Dyes (Fluorescence Video Microscopy)

Dyes

The use of intravital fluorescent dyes aims at the

— improvement of image contrast,

— visualization and morphometry of structures not detectable by conventional capillaroscopy,

— labeling of dynamic phenomena like transcapillary diffusion of small solutes or macromolecular permeability,

— evaluation of perfusion homogeneity and distinction between perfused and not perfused microvessels.

In clinical medicine, the available number of intravital dyes is limited to compounds that have been admitted for human use. Thus, many potentially helpful tracers (e.g., acridyl orange, FITC-labeled dextrans) cannot be injected intravenously. The exception is the local subepidermal application of minute amounts of FITC-dextran (fluorescence microlymphography; 3, 5).

To date, two fluorescent dyes have been introduced to study the microcirculation of skin or accessible mucosal layers: Na-fluorescein (NaF) and indocyanine green (ICG). Both were first used in ophthalmology, NaF for fluorescence angiography of the retina (49) and ICG for visualization of choroideal vessels (14, 15).

Because the small molecule NaF couples only partially to plasma proteins, it diffuses through the capillary wall even under physiologic conditions and stains the pericapillary interstitial space (2, 4, 29). The application of the dye opens the way to assess microvascular flow distribution, increased transcapillary and interstitial diffusion, and to study otherwise invisible areas like the pericapillary halo (2, 4, 6, 29, 42). ICG, which fluoresces in the near infrared, binds to plasma proteins in over 95% (39) and thus does not leave the intravascular compartment of healthy controls in detectable amounts (38).

Quantitative studies of fluorescent light intensities in different parts of the capillaroscopic image and at different times require the use of video systems. For analysis of the dynamic phenomena, video densitometers (1, 2, 4) or more recently computer-aided techniques of image processing (43) are essential.

The technique applying fluorescent tracers is called fluorescence video microscopy (2, 29). Essentially, the set-up consists of an incident-light fluorescence microscope equipped with appropriate filters, a sensitive video camera, a video tape recorder and instruments for optimizing video images and controlling the output of the lamp. The system is described in the following section, which is dedicated to NaF, and the necessary adaptations for ICG in the next chapter.

Although both dyes, NaF and ICG, have been used extensively with only exceptional side effects (9, 12, 47), precautions must be taken whenever the tracers are injected intravenously. A small indwelling catheter should be kept in place during the whole procedure. Appropriate medicaments counteracting allergic or pseudoallergic phenomena as well as a kit for resuscitation have to be ready for use. In patients presenting a history of allergic disease, caution is advised: Either the dyes should not be given at all, or special measures like previous administration of antiallergic drugs or corticosteroids should be considered. In any case, informed consent must be obtained from any patient. Pregnancy is a contraindication against the use of the fluorescent tracers.

Na-Fluorescein (NaF)

Fluorescence angiography of the retina is based on the intravenous application of NaF (49). This dye has also been used for evaluating distribution of skin flow on the macroscopic level (35), for testing viability of skin flaps, and for assessing gastric and duodenal mucosal blood flow (41). Geologists have colored lakes without superficial drainage by NaF in order to investigate underground water evacuation and connected sources.

At the microscopic level, NaF has been introduced to study microvascular flow distribution and transcapillary diffusion through the wall of single capillaries (2, 4, 29, 42) or in skin areas (1, 20). Unlike in retinal or cerebral microvessels, NaF diffuses out of the intravascular compartment under physiologic conditions and depicts a pericapillary space referred to as a halo. Increased transcapillary diffusion may only be diagnosed if diffusion of the tracer is increased in comparison to controls.

NaF has a molecular weight of 376 and is excreted mainly by the kidney. Patients should be instructed that their urine will show a green fluorescence for about one day.

The amount of the dye coupling to plasma proteins, especially albumin, has been reported to be about 40% (49). Recent detailed analyses revealed that 5 min after the injection, NaF circulates as a free compound in 15.2% of total NaF present in the plasma (31, 32). Two hours later, total NaF content of the plasma decreases to 0.6% of the value determined at 5 min. Unfortunately, there are no data about NaF concentration and the unbound portion early after dye administration.

NaF is injected into an antecubital vein as a bolus. Injection time should not exceed 2 s. 5–10 ml of physiologic saline solution are given immediately afterwards in order to enhance flow of dye toward the thoracic vessels. The dosage required for microvascular studies is relatively low and is adjusted according to the estimated individual blood volume (11). 0.2–0.3 ml/l estimated blood volume of a 20% solution are adequate for visualization of skin capillaries at any accessible part of the body (2, 6, 29, 42). 1–1.5 ml of 20% NaF are the dosages used in most instances.

NaF fluoresces in the visible part of the spectrum. A conventional fluorescence filter set with excitation at 450–500 nm and barrier at 515 nm is adequate (2, 18).

Nausea is the most common and harmless side effect of NaF. It manifests after about half a minute and is rarely the precursor of vomiting. Generalized itching and urticaria are uncommon, but may require administration of antihistaminics and possibly corticosteroids. The most serious side effect is hypotensive shock. The prevalence of severe reactions has been estimated to be about 0.4% (47). The necessity to leave a small indwelling catheter during the whole period of examination and to have available a resuscitation tray has been emphasized in the introductory part to fluorescence video microscopy.

Indocyanine Green (ICG)

ICG is a tricarbocyanine dye with a molecular weight of 775 developed originally for use as an indicator dye to determine circulation times in patients with intracardiac shunts (16, 17). It has subsequently been used in studies of hepatic function (8, 25, 37).

More recently, it was discovered that ICG fluorescing in the near infrared portion of the spectrum stains choroideal vessels previously inaccessible to in vivo studies (14, 15, 33). The technique has been found to be a valuable tool for the diagnosis of eye diseases such as choroideal tumors. As will be shown, the dye is also suitable to depict skin capillaries by infrared fluorescence video microscopy (38).

ICG leaves the circulation with a half-time of less than 10 min (37, 38). Plasma disappearance is biphasic showing a rapid initial phase with a half-time of 3–4 min and a later phase of slow elimination with a half-time of 68–88 min (37). It is completely excreted by the liver and minimally resorbed by the gastrointestinal tract (50).

Since the small molecular dye binds to plasma proteins in more than 95%, it circulates without a significant free component (39).

Figure 30 illustrates the spectral transmission characteristics of ICG and the properties of suitable excitation and barrier filters. ICG emits peak fluorescence at 835 nm. In this infrared portion of the spectrum, capillary filling by ICG

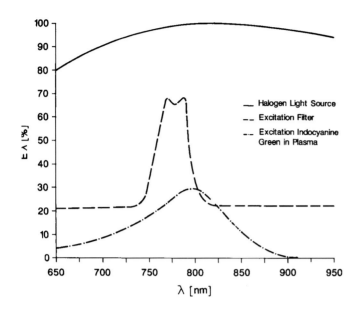

Figure 30.
(a) Spectral transmission characteristics: Excitation curve of indocyanine green (ICG) in plasma, halogen or Xenon light source, and excitation filter.

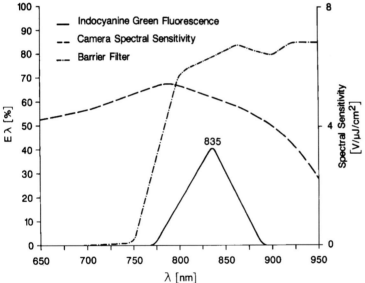

(b) Spectral transmission characteristics of ICG fluorescence in whole blood, spectral sensitivity of a microchip TV camera (Krantz), and barrier filter.

escapes to visual observation. An infrared sensitive video camera is used to detect the dye.

In the first studies performed, dosage of ICG was 50 mg/l of estimated individual blood volume (38). As has recently been demonstrated (unpublished data), a lower dosage yields comparable results. 25 mg/l or 100–125 mg in patients with normal weight are now used routinely and should be preferred to the higher amounts injected previously. The viscous fluid is given within 5–10 s and is followed by an appropriate amount of physiologic saline solution.

ICG is of proven safety with only rare serious adverse effects in widespread clinical use (9). Exceptionally, allergic or pseudoallergic

Figure 31. Recording system for fluorescence video microscopy.

(a) Setup with intravital microscope mounted on a heavy support and a flexible arm, DC power supply, TV camera, video screen, and tape recorder. The cathode-ray oscilloscope below the monitor serves to improve the video images, the photometer to control the output of the mercury vapor lamp.

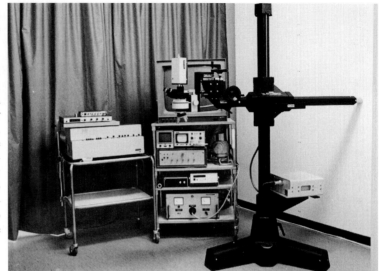

(b) Microscope with TV camera. The system of screws allows perfect adaptation to the skin surface.

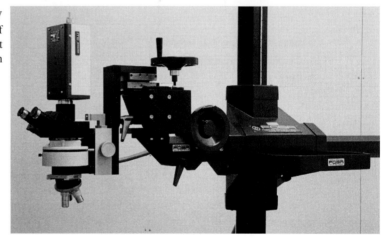

phenomena occur including hypotensive shock. Disease states with pathologic plasma proteins seem to be particularly subject to complications. These patients should be excluded from ICG studies. The necessary prophylactic measures have been described above.

System for Fluorescence Video Microscopy

Essentially, the system used for intravital fluorescence video microscopy consists of a recording (**Figure 31**) and an evaluation unit. Data are collected through the intact skin by a fluorescence microscope with epi-illumination and a video system. They are analyzed by different techniques of densitometry. Without interposed fluorescent filters, the system is also suited to perform conventional capillaroscopy and measurement of red blood cell velocity.

Recording Unit

The *fluorescence microscope* (2, 6, 18, 29, 42) works with epi-illumination (Wild-Leitz). Light

Dynamic Capillaroscopy with Dyes (Fluorescence Video Microscopy)

is provided by a 100 W mercury vapor lamp (conventional capillaroscopy, velocity measurements, NaF studies) or by a 100 W Xenon lamp (ICG), directed to the skin surface through the optical system of the microscope. A heat absorption filter (KG1, Wild-Leitz) and a blue filter (BG 7) for contrast enhancement are interposed between lamp and microscope. The light source is connected to a DC-power supply (Irem).

In order to avoid disturbing reflections from the skin, the incident illuminator is equipped with a "pol-cube" (Wild-Leitz) consisting of a mirror with 50% reflectance and 50% transmittance, placed at 45° to the optical axis of the microscope, in combination with a polarizer and an analyzer (46). **Figure 32** illustrates how the "pol-cube" improves image quality.

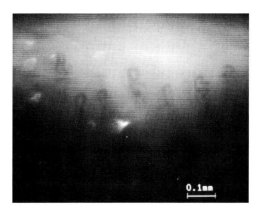

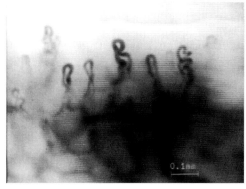

Figure 32. Capillaroscopic image without (above) and with (below) the use of a "pol-cube" to avoid light reflections. (Reprinted with permission from Slaaf et al., 46)

Depending on the purpose of the study, different objectives are used: plan 2.5/0.08, plan fluotar 6.3/0.20 or 10/0.25 (Wild-Leitz). The corresponding magnifications on a television screen with a diagonal diameter of 42 cm are 81×, 200×, and 310×, respectively. The magnification may be increased by the use of other lenses or larger monitors up to about 700–800×. The smaller magnifications are selected for an overview, for evaluation of microvascular flow distribution, and for measurement of transcapillary diffusion in skin areas (1, 19, 20). Detailed studies of single capillary loops require large magnifications.

The working distance of the objectives exceeds 6 mm. It allows microinjections in the field of observation or the placement of special probes for determination of transcutaneous oxygen tension or of laser Doppler flux (see page 60).

For studies with NaF the *fluorescence filter set* comprises an excitation filter operating at 450–490 nm and a barrier filter at 515 nm (2, 29). The values for ICG are 750–800 nm and 750 nm, respectively (38). The ICG filters are provided by Ditric Optics. After having localized the capillaries to be studied by conventional capillaroscopy, the filters are inserted by a switch mechanism just after intravenous injection of the dye.

Optimal adaptation of the microscope to the skin area under study and sufficient stability of the system are obtained by a heavy *support* (Foba, **Figure 31b**). A horizontal arm carrying the microscope may be moved three-dimensionally (Wild-Leitz). Coarse adjustment is performed by wheels, fine adjustment by micrometer screws.

A sensitive *television camera* (e.g., Cadmium Selenide Vidicon®, Siemens) is mounted on the microscope. Its peak sensitivity should correspond to the nanometer range of fluorescence emission. Whereas normal cameras are adequate for recording NaF images, ICG fluorescing in the near infrared requires cameras still adequately sensitive around 835 nm (38). So far, microchip devices have been used for ICG with the specifications given in **Figure 30**.

The automatic control of the light level is disconnected for measurements of transcapillary diffusion (densitometry), but may be of value for obtaining optimal images whenever morphology is the only purpose of the study. A switch mechanism for selecting one of the two possibilities is useful.

The dynamic visual information gained by the camera is transmitted to a *monitor* and a *video tape recorder*. In previous studies tape recorders with a tape width of 1 inch (BK 204, Grundig) were preferred (1, 2, 6, 29), since traditionally they were the only ones with adequate optical resolution and automatized display of single frames. Recently, however, advancement in television technology has made it possible to use much less expensive machines with smaller tape diameters.

It is convenient to use a *video timer and scale marker* (For-A Company). Date of investigation, running time after dye injection, and scale appear on the video screen.

Additional devices complete the video microscopy system (6). They are only necessary for quantitative measurements of fluorescent light intensity (densitometry). A cathode ray oscilloscope helps to improve the quality of the television recordings. The output of the lamp is controlled by a photometer before and after each measurement of transcapillary diffusion in order to recognize sudden loss of power. Moreover, fluorescent light intensity may be standardized according to the mean light intensity level observed in a set of investigations.

Procedure

Controls or patients are examined in supine position, though measurements in sitting position are also possible (20). The finger with best skin transparency or with the most characteristic findings is placed below the microscope and fixed by plasticine. When the study is performed on the lower leg or the foot, a vacuum pillow is used to fix the extremity. Depending on the skin region explored, patients rest on the right or left side (medial ankle) or lie on their backs with slightly flexed knee (dorsum of the foot, toes).

At least 20 min are allowed to elapse until the fluorochromes are injected as a bolus. Room temperature should be comfortable between 20–24°C.

A drop of paraffin oil improves skin transparency. First, the capillaries are visualized at low magnification without insertion of fluorescent filters. The single capillary or the skin area is selected for study, and magnification is adjusted to the corresponding requirements. A small indwelling catheter is placed in an antecubital vein and kept in place during the whole procedure.

NaF or ICG are injected as a bolus with the dosage described above. Before switching to the fluorescent filter set, the capillaries are focused again. Whereas the microvessels may be still recognized as shadows after insertion of the NaF filters, no picture is obtained after insertion of the ICG filters until the dye fluorescing in the near infrared reaches the capillary loops. Rapid refocusing is essential. If both fluorochromes are to be applied during the same study, ICG is injected first because of its shorter elimination half-time.

As outlined in the method critique, transcapillary diffusion of small solutes like NaF varies with flow rate (26). Since it is not feasible to adjust blood flow of a skin area to identical levels in different subjects or patients, an effort to control temperature is essential. For this purpose, a finger cuff is placed around the proximal phalanx and connected to a thermostat (4). Water temperature is then adjusted to a somewhat higher degree (2–3°C) than the skin temperature desired in the area of measurement. The latter is monitored by a skin thermometer or a thermocouple providing a continuous reading. The adequate temperatures at the finger tip vary between 28° and 30°C.

At the foot, the skin is cooled or warmed up by a cold pack (3M) or a heating pad wrapped around the ankle (1). A skin temperature of 30°C at the foot dorsum and 31°C at the medial ankle appears to be adequate.

Data Processing

Morphometric and dynamic data are analyzed off-line by replay of the information stored on the video tape. Fluorescent light intensity in defined areas may also be processed on-line. The various techniques used for evaluating the quantitative data include direct measurements on the television screen, image shearing, and video densitometry. Recently, multipurpose video image analysis using personal computers has increasingly replaced the older methods designed for single applications (34, 43).

Image Enhancement

Certain images obtained by intravital fluorescence microscopy do not contain sufficient optical resolution for proper analysis. Especially ICG emits fluorescence with low intensity requiring improvement of contrast. **Figure 33** gives an example of a capillary loop depicted by ICG before and after image enhancement.

An elegant technique for enhancing contrast is nonlinear amplification of gray levels contained in the video image (27). Image subtraction also improves the quality of television pictures.

Appearance Time

The time interval between the end of tracer injection and first arrival in the field of observation is called the appearance time. It is best determined by the use of a video timer indicating the running time started after the end of dye injection. A stopwatch may also be used.

The time elapsing between filling of the first and last capillaries visualized in a given field is also determined. In most cases, not all the microvessels begin to fluoresce at the same time. This interval is a measure for homogeneity of microvascular perfusion and depends either on the functional condition of the arterioles or on rheological factors, especially in low flow states.

Measurement of Diameters and Areas

The diameters of microvessels can often be determined on single frames of television recordings by direct caliber measurement on the video monitor. Since it is difficult even for a trained observer to determine vessel diameters by manual evaluation, the result depends to a certain degree on subjective decisions. Still more cumbersome are measurements of areas requiring the use of planimeters.

Image-shearing monitors solve the problem in part but require a special set-up. Diameters may also be traced on the video screen with the mouse of a personal computer. Automatized read-out of the values is provided for a given magnification (22, 43). This technique, included in a multipurpose image analysis system, is the most useful one for area measurements

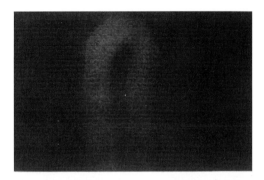
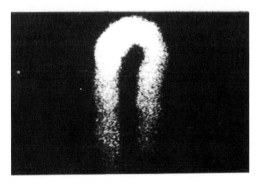

Figure 33. Image of a nailfold capillary filled with ICG before (above) and after (below) image enhancement by a computerized image-analysis system (nonlinear amplification of grey levels).

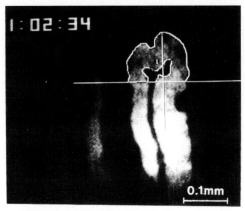

area: $9.22 \cdot 10^{-3}$ mm^2

Figure 34. Measurements of microvascular areas. (a) Enlarged nailfold capillary loop of a patient with progressive systemic sclerosis depicted by ICG. The area of the loop apex is measured distal of a line defined at 100 µm from the apex.

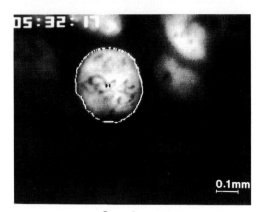

area: $6.29 \cdot 10^{-2}$ mm^2

(b) Measurement of halo area at the medial ankle in a patient with chronic venous insufficiency. The halo containing a meandering capillary loop is stained by NaF.

(**Figure 34**). Promising for the future is automatic diameter tracing (43) or measurement of microvessel length (10).

With both ICG and NaF as fluorescent tracers it became possible to determine four microvascular dimensions at the nailfold (7): red cell column (conventional capillaroscopy), full

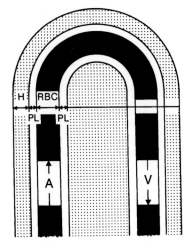

■ Red cell column (RBC)   ☐ Plasma layer (PL)
▦ Halo (H)

Figure 35. Schematic drawing of a nailfold capillary loop with four microvascular compartments. The capillary diameter comprises the width of red blood cell column (RBC) and of plasma layer (PL) on both sides. H = pericapillary halo, A = arterial limb of the loop, V = venous limb.

capillary diameter (ICG), plasma layer (ICG), and pericapillary halo (NaF). These four compartments are shown in **Figure 35**.

The plasma layer on both sides of the erythrocyte column is easily calculated by subtracting red cell column width (RBC) from diameter of full capillary (D). A direct determination on ICG pictures is not possible because of insufficient visualization of red blood cell column in the presence of ICG.

NaF images may be used to estimate halo diameters (see also page 45, Table 7). Since the erythrocyte column is well visible on the NaF recordings, it is easy to determine the distance (M) between the outer border of the erythrocyte column and the outer limit of the pericapillary halo stained by NaF (**Figure 35**). This distance comprises the external part of the plasma layer and the pericapillary halo. The approximate halo diameter (H) may be calculated by the equation

Dynamic Capillaroscopy with Dyes (Fluorescence Video Microscopy)

$$H = M - \frac{(D - RBC)}{2}.$$

It is assumed that the plasma layer (PL) is equally distributed on the inner and outer side of the hair-pin shaped capillary loop. This hypothesis appears to be reasonably adequate for the straight parts of the arterial and venous capillary limb but may be questionable at the loop apex (7).

Densitometry

Intra- and pericapillary fluorescent light intensities are measured by video densitometers. They reflect the amount of dye present in the area examined. By evaluating fluorescent light intensities just outside the capillary wall, transcapillary diffusion through the wall is quantified. High fluorescent light intensities correspond to high transcapillary diffusion and vice versa. Measurements in a different compartment (e.g., inside and outside the pericapillary halo) are suited to assess complex diffusion patterns.

It must be realized that the light intensity values obtained are not identical with exact concentrations of the fluorochrome. Different factors influence the readings, including light transmission properties of the skin, scattering of reflected fluorescent light, and irradiation from deeper invisible layers. Because of the considerable interindividual variation of these factors, diffusion coefficients or surface area products cannot be determined.

Fluorescent light intensities are expressed in arbitrary units or in percent of the individual maximal light intensity reached during the investigation (1, 2, 18, 20). The first procedure is preferred for comparative measurements in identical subjects or patients in whom skin properties are reasonably constant. The best example is the testing of therapeutic effects, where intraindividual changes are evaluated. For comparison between different groups, for example, between healthy controls and long-term diabetics, the second interindividual procedure is best suited. When the values are expressed as a percentage of the individual maximal fluorescent light intensity, differing properties of the skin are of no major importance. Spontaneous fluorescence of the skin serves as baseline (zero) and not the black level of the video camera.

The *conventional setup for video densitometry* (1, 2, 4, 6, 18, 29) includes monitor, densitometer (IPM, Colorado Video), xy-plotter, and strip-chart recorder (**Figure 36**). For recording light intensities on lines crossing single capillary loops or several adjacent loops, a single

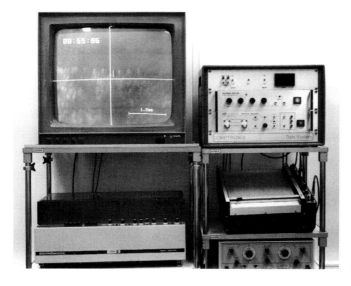

Figure 36. System for video densitometry composed of tape recorder, TV monitor, video densitometer, and xy-plotter.

frame of the video tape is displayed on the monitor. The densitometer line is projected onto the screen and placed with respect to the capillary to be studied. A point or a small window is moved on the axis. The light intensities are recorded by the xy-plotter as a two-dimensional curve (**Figure 37**).

Defined anatomical sites are selected for measuring fluorescent light intensity (see below). The measurements are performed on the tracings using arbitrary units. The level of spontaneous skin fluorescence established before dye arrival serves as baseline. For calculating percentage values, the highest value encountered during the recording period is considered to be 100%.

Systems for image analysis are currently introduced for video densitometry and will probably replace conventional techniques (43). Frames of the television recording are digitized and displayed on the monitor. Lines for densitometry are placed by means of a personal computer and sites of measurement selected (**Figure 38**). Without any further manipulation, the computer is told to plot densitometer curves and to print fluorescent light intensities at the chosen sites of measurement. Values in percent of individual maximal light intensity are calculated automatically.

For clinical studies, *three main techniques of densitometry* solving different problems have been used (6):

— line densitometry at the single capillary level,

— line densitometry encompassing several or multiple adjacent loops, and

— densitometry in rectangular areas containing a larger number of capillaries ("large window technique").

Line Densitometry at the Single Capillary Level

For detailed analysis of fluorescent light intensity distribution around a selected capillary loop, the nailfold area of fingers or toes is suited best (2, 4, 6, 29). Large magnifications are

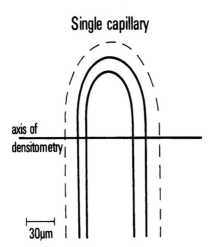
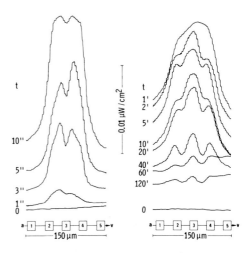

Figure 37. Video densitometry of single capillary loops.
Left: Horizontal axis of densitometry crossing the arterial and venous limb of the capillary loop, the pericapillary halo on both sides, and the remote interstitial space outside the halo boundary.
Right: Densitometer curves recorded on this axis at different times after arrival of the fluorescent dye NaF in a healthy volunteer. The tracings with two peaks correspond to the filling phase of the two limbs, the tracings with three peaks to later times when the most intensive fluorescence emanates from the pericapillary halo and the space between the capillary loop limbs. The steep descending part of the curve is located at the halo border. The numbers 1–5 indicate sites of measurement frequently used.

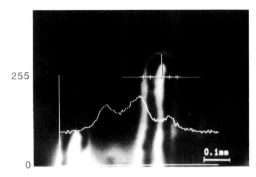

Figure 38. Video densitometry by computer-aided image analysis. After designation of the nailfold capillary apex by the mouse (arrow), the densitometer line is automatically drawn at a distance of 100 µm, and the densitometer curve is displayed on the screen. The sites selected for measurement of fluorescence light intensity are indicated. The values may be printed in arbitrary units or in percent of the individual maximum value.

needed. A line running perpendicular to the arterial and venous limb at a defined distance from the apex has been used in most studies (**Figures 37** and **38**; 2, 29). The distance commonly selected is 33 µm. For special purposes, any other axis for densitometry may be projected on the television monitor. Longitudinal lines of measurement have been placed parallel to capillary loops on the arterial and venous side (2). For analysis of diffusion at the apex, a line running between the two limbs and crossing the vertex of the loop into the distal interstitial space is used.

The interesting sites of measurement for evaluating transcapillary and interstitial diffusion of NaF are located on the arterial or venous limb of the capillary, within the pericapillary halo and outside of it (see **Figure 35**). They are defined and transferred to the densitometer tracing. A distance of 6–8 µm from the external border of the red blood cell column is convenient for intrahalo measurements, a distance of 40 µm (32–34 µm from the intrahalo site) for determination outside the halo boundary. In enlarged loops with increased width of the plasma layer, the measuring site within the halo should be about 10 µm outside the outer border of the erythrocyte column. Especially at the apex, where enlarged halos may be observed, does the site of measurement outside the halo limit have to be displaced in distal direction.

The determinations are repeated several times after first appearance of the fluorochrome in the capillary selected for study. Times used frequently are 3, 5, 10, 20, 30, 40, and 50 s, and 1, 2, 3, 4, 5, 10, 20, and 30 min.

Line Densitometry Encompassing Several Capillaries

The homogeneity of microvascular perfusion (19) or diffusion into avascular areas (6) may be analyzed by this technique (**Figure 39**); relatively low magnifications are used. Capillaries filled by the fluorescent dye produce a single peak of light intensity without pericapillary details. A three-dimensional arrangement of tracings recorded at different times allows an overview of homogeneous or inhomogeneous microvascular perfusion (see **Figure 57**, page 70) and of tracer diffusion into avascular fields (see **Figure 75**, page 100).

The position of the axis is selected according to the problem to be solved. For studying avascular areas, the densitometer line runs perpendicular to the border of the field. If homogeneity of perfusion is tested, the axis is positioned crossing various capillaries arranged in a row on the densitometer line (**Figure 39**). A fluorescent light intensity peak appears at the time of dye filling. Large time intervals between the filling of individual loops is characteristic for inhomogeneous perfusion, almost simultaneous filling for homogeneous perfusion (see page 46).

Densitometry in Rectangular Areas

Line densitometry across single capillary loops has the advantage of excellent spatial resolution. Light intensity differences in various capillary and pericapillary compartments may be analyzed. However, transcapillary diffusion may vary among adjacent capillaries. Densitometry in window-shaped fields (**Figure 40**) yields more representative values for skin areas.

Figure 40.
Above: Tracing obtained in a normal subject. The ascending curve corresponds to rising intensity of fluorescent light in the area covered by the window-shaped densitometer.

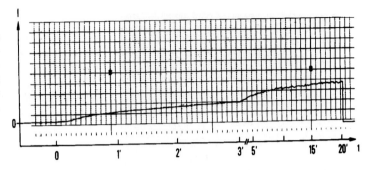

Below: Window densitometry in a defined quadratic or rectangular skin area. The points represent capillary loops appearing as dots (dorsum of the foot, medial ankle).

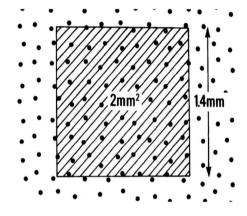

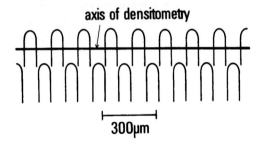

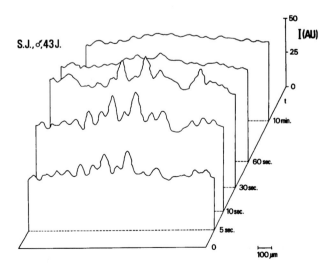

Figure 39. Line densitometry for evaluation of microvascular flow distribution.
Above: Densitometer line crossing a number of schematically drawn capillary loops.
Below: Densitometer tracings at different times after NaF appearance at the nailfold in a healthy volunteer. The small peaks of fluorescent light intensity correspond to single capillary loops that are almost simultaneously filled by the dye.

Dynamic Capillaroscopy with Dyes (Fluorescence Video Microscopy)

The technique is easily applied in any suitable part of the body like the dorsum of the foot (1, 20) or the medial ankle region (6). For this method it does not matter whether capillary loops are arranged parallel to the skin surface or whether they emerge from below. One should count the number of capillary loops included in the rectangular field before and after appearance of the dye. On-line densitometer curves are recorded on chart-strip (**Figure 40**). Off-line evaluation during the playback of video recordings is also possible. Like at the sites defined on single capillary tracings, fluorescent light intensity may be measured at different times.

Evaluation and Critique

Figure 41 shows how the use of NaF may improve detection of perfused capillaries. In a white scar from irradiation 20 years ago only a few microvessels were visualized with conventional capillaroscopy. A much more detailed image was obtained after filling the capillaries and venules with NaF. Many microvessels were invisible at the analysis with white light but clearly depicted by the fluorescent dye.

The *linearity* of each video densitometry system should be checked from time to time. A test signal generator (Tektronix) producing known steps of light intensity or a set of tubes containing different known concentrations of the dye may be used (2, 29). The results of such an evaluation are shown in **Figure 42**.

The influence of *fluorescence fading* has been tested with cuvettes containing different concentrations of NaF (2). Fading becomes more relevant with increasing concentrations. During exposure to the light of a 100 W mercury vapor lamp below the microscope lasting 20 min, light intensity decreased by 4% in a tube emitting 0.32 µW/cm² of light intensity. Since the fluorescent light intensity frequently occurring in intravital studies is inferior to 0.20 µW/cm², the error induced by fluorescence fading should not exceed 2–3%.

It has recently been demonstrated (44) that continuous illumination of microvessels filled by fluorescent dyes in experimental animals induces increased macromolecular permeability

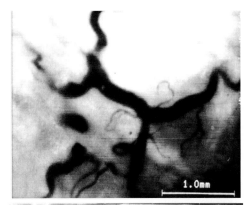

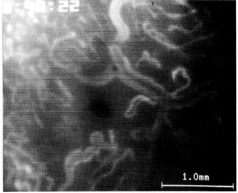

Figure 41. Skin microvessels in a scar at the lower leg after local irradiation 20 years previously.
Above: Conventional capillaroscopy. Apparently, there is marked reduction of the number of capillaries.
Below: Fluorescence video microscopy after injection of NaF. Many more microvessels are now visualized after dye application.

after exposures lasting more than 10 min. This effect is lacking when intermittent exposures lasting 15 s are used. No comparable data are available for transcapillary diffusion of small solutes in humans. However, the most important values for transcapillary diffusion of NaF are gained within the first 5 min after dye arrival.

Transcapillary diffusion of small solutes depends not only on capillary wall properties, but also on capillary flow (26). In previous studies, care was taken that flow velocities in the control and patient group were not significantly different (4), or that flow velocity was lower in

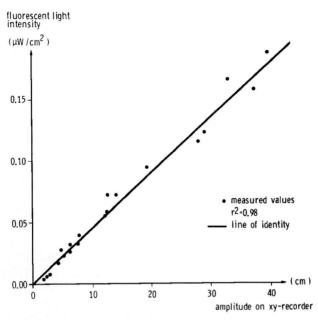

Figure 42. Measured and expected values of fluorescent light intensity emanating from 10 cuvettes with known NaF concentrations (0.001–0.05 mg/100 mg). The input into the videocamera was measured by a power meter adapted to the camera piece of the microscope ($\mu W/cm^2$), the amplitudes by the video densitometer system on the xy-recorder.

the patients although they exhibited increased diffusion. An accurate control of temperature as described in the chapter "Procedure" (page 36) helps to standardize flow conditions (1, 4). In future investigations, the exact correlations between flow and diffusion have to be established on the capillary level (velocity measurements) and in skin areas (comparison to laser Doppler data). Problems arising from using different dye brands are mentioned further below.

Normal Microvascular Dimensions

The different microvascular dimensions accessible to measurement (see page 38 and **Figure 35**) include diameter of capillary, red blood cell column, plasma layer, and pericapillary halo. By conventional capillaroscopy without the use of fluorescent dyes, it is only possible to determine the width of the red blood cell column, which is often referred to as "capillary diameter." In fact, the real capillary diameter includes red blood cell column and plasma layer. The combination of conventional capil-

laroscopy and indocyanine green technique (7, 38) or the intraarterial injection of FITC-labeled albumin (36) permits calculation of plasma layer dimensions. The latter may vary widely with flow velocity (21). After a capillary flow stop, the erythrocytes accelerate and often leave an empty loop for a short period of time. Therefore, diameters of plasma layer should be measured at defined flow velocities especially for group comparison. When fluorescence video microscopy with NaF is performed in addition to the ICG method, the halo dimensions may also be determined (7).

The nailfold capillaries are larger than other capillaries of the body, which often require deformation of circulating single erythrocytes. In most instances erythrocytes form a column when passing through the nailfold loops.

The width of the *erythrocyte column* (RBC) is well known. **Table 7** contains the mean values measured in three studies (7, 28, 36). They are well comparable. RBC column is largest at the apex of the loop and smallest at the arterial limb.

The mean values indicated in **Table 7** are the only ones reported in the literature for all the four microvascular dimensions. By injecting

Table 7. Mean normal diameters and standard deviations (μm) of capillary (D), red cell column (RBC), plasma layer (PL), and halo (H) (Brülisauer & Bollinger, 7).

	Arterial limb	Apex	Venous limb
D	17.7 ± 3.6	29.4 ± 4.2	20.4 ± 3.7
	15.0 ± 2.5*		16.7 ± 3.0*
RBC	12.3 ± 2.9	18.5 ± 5.4	13.5 ± 3.5
	10.8 ± 3.0*		12.1 ± 2.7*
	12.9 ± 1.0**	16.9 ± 2.1**	15.8 ± 1.8**
PL	5.4 ± 2.4	10.9 ± 5.8	6.9 ± 2.9
	4.2 ± 0.7*		4.6 ± 0.8*
H	8.3 ± 4.5	9.0 ± 5.8	8.0 ± 4.1

* values measured by Mahler et al. (36) before and after intraarterial injection of FITC-tagged albumin

** values determined by Jacobs et al. (28) by conventional capillaroscopy

FITC-tagged albumin into the cubital artery, similar values were measured for the width of capillary, red cell column, and *plasma layer*. The fact that the plasma layer is in direct contact with the capillary wall is also called plasma skimming or Fåhraeus-Lindqvist effect (13). On both the arterial and venous part of nailfold capillary loops plasma occupies about 32% of full capillary limb diameter (38; **Figure 43**). Arterial limb diameter of the capillary averaged 17.7 ± 3.6 μm and erythrocyte column width 12.3 ± 2.9 μm. By subtraction of the two values, a mean plasma layer diameter of 5.4 ± 2.4 μm was calculated. Again, apex diameters were larger than arterial and venous limb diameters. These values were determined with normal flow velocity without marked fluctuations of corpuscular speed.

No comparative values to the ones given in **Table 7** are available for *halo diameters* (see **Figure 35** and **Figure 45**). This compartment extends about 8 μm outside both the arterial and venous limb of nailfold capillary loops (7). Under physiologic conditions, mean halo diameter is not significantly larger at the apex than at the two loop limbs (9.0 ± 5.8 μm).

Halo diameters also have be determined at the medial ankle region (23, 45). The values averaged 81 ± 15 μm in healthy controls (23); slightly lower mean values were measured by Saner and co-workers (45). These values represent diameters of the entire pericapillary matrix in which the loops are embedded (see **Figure 34**). Thus, they cannot be compared to those measured at the nailfold where the halo next to the arterial, apical and venous part of the capillary wall has been determined (**Table 7**). The ankle values correspond to the sum of halo diameters on both sides, both capillary limb diameters and the distance between the two limbs.

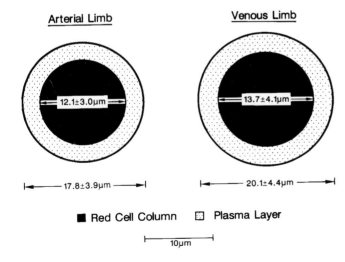

Figure 43. Mean diameter of capillary (red blood cell column and plasma layer) and red cell column in 29 capillaries of 11 healthy subjects (38).

The halo region has not been fully explored by electron microscopy. It seems to correspond to a perivascular matrix described by Higgins and Eady (24). This compartment contains pericytes, mast cells, and collagen fibrils. Oedland (40) found concentric collagen lamellae in the pericapillary region.

Appearance Time

Appearance time—the time elapsing between the end of dye injection and appearance at the site of measurement—is composed of the circulation time through the veins to the heart, the lungs, the large and small arteries. Since main vascular resistance is located at the arterioles, varying circulation times essentially depend on the function of precapillary vessels.

Different appearance times have been described in the literature according to the mode of dye application. The shortest mean appearance times are obtained by elevation of the arm after injection or by injection during reactive hyperemia after arterial occlusion (35). Somewhat longer times are observed without manipulation. It must be realized that during intravital capillaroscopy the skin section to be examined has to be kept as motionless as possible. Any maneuvers may induce movement artefacts. Therefore, most authors prefer injecting the dye without elevating the arm or performing reactive hyperemia. A bolus of physiological saline solution following dye injection does not interfere with optimal fixation and is advised.

In **Table 8**, mean normal values and ranges of appearance times are given for the nailfold and the dorsum of the foot. As expected, the former are shorter than the latter: Without manipulation a typical appearance time at the nailfold is about 30 s and at the foot dorsum about 55 s. The upper normal limit at the nailfold is 50 s, at the foot 90 s.

In one of the nailfold studies, a relatively high mean value (47.6 ± 16.8) was recorded in healthy subjects (38). This value is mostly due to one extremely long appearance time (80 s). Moreover, this study was performed with ICG

Table 8. Mean appearance time (a) and time between first dye appearance and filling of all capillaries (b) (range).

Authors	Nailfold	
	(a)	(b)
Bollinger et al. (2)	34.6 ± 7.2 s (25–45 s)	
Franzeck et al. (19)	27.6 ± 6.1 s (20–42 s)	10 s
Moneta et al. (38)	47.6 ± 16.8 s (22–80 s)	

Authors	Dorsum of the foot	
	(a)	(b)
Jünger et al. (30)	53.4 ± 15.7 s (23–82 s)	23.2 ± 7.6 s (12–48 s)
Baer & Bollinger (1)	55.8 ± 14.8 s (27–90 s)	34.0 ± 11.2 s (17–50 s)

that is more difficult to inject quickly because of the relatively viscous dye solution. The author once observed a dye appearance time of more than 4 min in a young medical doctor who was afraid of the injection. Generalized vasoconstriction is the main cause of prolonged circulation times measured occasionally in normals.

Microvascular Flow Distribution

The time interval between arrival of the dye in the first capillaries visualized and the last ones filled by the dye is a simple and reliable parameter for testing the homogeneity of microvascular perfusion. At the nailfold, all capillaries are stained by NaF within 12 s (19), and longer time intervals indicate inhomogeneous flow distribution. As shown elsewhere (page 42), line densitometry performed at consecutive times is a way to document the homogeneity or inhomogeneity of microvascular flow. Homogeneous flow in a given field of observation is characterized by simultaneous or almost simultaneous peaks of fluorescent light intensity corresponding to single microvessels (see **Figure 39**).

The time interval is much longer at the dorsum of the foot (**Table 8**). Inhomogeneity of

Dynamic Capillaroscopy with Dyes (Fluorescence Video Microscopy)

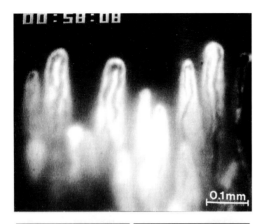

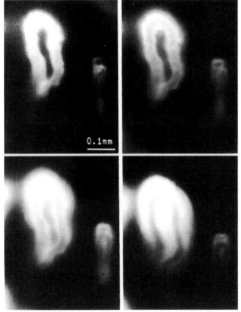

Figure 44.
Above: Image taken from the TV monitor 25 s after NaF appearance at the nailfold (58 s after dye injection). Bright filling of the pericapillary halo with well-delineated outer border (control subject).
Below: Diffusion of NaF through the nailfold capillary wall with filling of the pericapillary halo (patient with scleroderma) 4 s after dye appearance (top left): the capillary wall is outlined but already a bit blurred; 10 s (top right) and 14 s (bottom left): filling of the halo; 24 s (bottom right): the outer border of the halo is now well depicted, the red blood cells appear as a dark column, the microvessel wall is not delineated.

dye inflow may be diagnosed if more than 50 s elapse between first and last capillary filling within the observation field (1).

There are two potential main reasons for inhomogeneous microvascular flow: vasospasm at the level of the invisible feeding arterioles or hemorheological changes. Through intravital capillaroscopy it is not possible to decide which of the two mechanisms is involved.

Transcapillary and Interstitial Diffusion of NaF

Diffusion Pattern in Normal Subjects

Immediately after reaching the capillary loops at the nailfold, NaF diffuses through the capillary wall and depicts a pericapillary compartment called halo (**Figure 44**; 2, 4, 29, 42). The capillary wall is not visualized accurately, whereas the outer border of the halo is delineated and remains visible for as long as 10–20 min. The compartment outside of the halo limit emits much less fluorescent light than the halo region itself. The most intensive fluorescence emanates from the area between the two limbs of the capillary loop. Transcapillary diffusion of the dye appears to be symmetrical with respect to the loop and without preferential sites of dye passage. Outside the halo border, NaF does not accumulate in cloud- or street-like areas.

Later, after dye arrival, the red blood cells appear as a central black column (**Figure 44**). The capillary wall is not well delineated. The distance between the outer border of the erythrocyte column and the halo boundary is composed of plasma layer and halo diameter (see **Figure 35**).

Using special oil-immersion objectives for detection of fluorescent light (NPL Fluotar® 25/0.75, Wild-Leitz), the optical resolution may be optimized, the vessel wall and halo configuration depicted precisely by NaF alone (**Figure 45**). However, these objectives should not be applied for determination of transcapillary diffusion, because skin compression is likely to

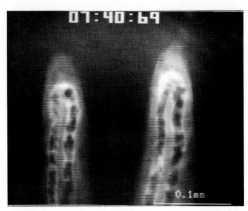

Figure 45. Nailfold capillary loops 52 s after NaF arrival in a patient with rheumatoid arthritis. A special fluorescence objective with oil immersion (Wild-Leitz) was used. The intravascular compartment fluoresces brightly and contains dark flowing erythrocytes. Vessel wall and outer border of pericapillary halo are both depicted by NaF alone.

occur and to alter microvascular hemodynamics.

In other skin regions where the capillaries do not run parallel to the skin surface and their apex appears as dot or comma, the pericapillary halo is also rapidly stained. It has a circular aspect (see **Figure 34b**). This configuration has been observed at the dorsum of the foot (1) and at the medial ankle (23, 45). Like at the nailfold, the remote interstitial space contains less dye than the pericapillary halo. A mesh-like arrangement of skin capillaries was occasionally found in the ankle region (23). When this particular anatomic pattern is present, the otherwise typical circular halos are lacking or atypical.

Densitometer Curves

Immediately after NaF reaches the capillary loops under study, the distribution of fluorescent light intensity on a line crossing the arterial and venous limb of a single capillary loop (nailfold) is first characterized by two peaks corresponding to the dye just arriving at the two limbs. This period is very short. The prompt transcapillary diffusion of NaF and the filling of the pericapillary halo then produce a tracing with three peaks corresponding to the halo region on both sides of the loop and to the area between the two limbs (see **Figures 37** and **38**; 2, 4, 29, 42).

Fluorescent light intensity decreases steeply at the halo border. It is high within the halo and low outside of it. The steep gradient of light intensity is maintained for 10–20 min and does not change location (see **Figure 37**). This indicates that a physiologic diffusion barrier is effective at the outer limit of the halo.

If densitometry is performed in skin areas by the "large window technique," on-line densitometer tracings reflect the increase of fluorescent light intensity in this region containing a certain number of capillaries (see **Figure 40**; 1, 20). A flat slope documents slow accumulation of the fluorescent material in the interstitial space, a steep ascending slope fast accumulation.

Normal Values of Pericapillary and Interstitial Fluorescent Light Intensity

At the *single capillary level*, fluorescent light intensity has been determined at various time intervals from first dye appearance inside and outside the pericapillary halo. Sites of measurement have to be defined precisely with respect to the capillary loop (see page 40).

The mean values measured in two studies (2, 4) are given in **Table 9**. There were significant differences of fluorescent light intensity ($p<0.001$) between the halo and the more remote compartment up to 10 or 20 min, suggesting that the halo border acts as a barrier for diffusion. An alternative explanation would involve coupling of NaF to interstitial molecules within the pericapillary halo (2, 4).

There are no significant intraindividual differences of fluorescent light intensity inside the halo near the arterial and venous limb of the capillary loop. NaF diffuses in equal amounts through the wall of both limbs. In other words, transcapillary diffusion of small molecular NaF is symmetrical with respect to the arterial and venous side of the loop (2, 4, 29).

Dynamic Capillaroscopy with Dyes (Fluorescence Video Microscopy)

Table 9. Fluorescent light intensities on the arterial side of nailfold capillary loops in percent of maximum individual light intensity.

Reference	% inside halo		% outside halo	
	(2)	(4)	(2)	(4)
3 s	17.8 ± 11.9	15.2 ± 5.5	12.7 ± 10.5	8.3 ± 3.8
10 s	42.9 ± 19.2	43.3 ± 20.7	26.0 ± 12.9	22.6 ± 11.9
30 s	69.0 ± 9.9	61.4 ± 12.2	46.9 ± 11.0	39.0 ± 12.1
1 min	70.3 ± 12.5	65.4 ± 10.1	52.2 ± 10.5	46.0 ± 10.7
10 min	54.1 ± 15.6	48.3 ± 20.7	48.7 ± 14.6	43.1 ± 18.3
20 min	41.6 ± 14.6	33.9 ± 15.4	39.4 ± 13.5	29.6 ± 13.6

Table 10. Mean fluorescent light intensity (in % of maximum individual values) at the dorsum of the foot (proximal to basis of first and second toe) and at the medial ankle in normal controls.

Reference	(1)*	(30)*	(23)**
3 s	—	1.8 ± 2.1	2.2 ± 1.9
10 s	8.2 ± 5.3	3.9 ± 3.6	5.9 ± 5.0
30 s	21.1 ± 7.6	11.6 ± 6.5	14.7 ± 9.0
1 min	36.2 ± 6.8	20.4 ± 7.4	23.6 ± 11.1
5 min	77.4 ± 5.9	66.0 ± 11.9	62.6 ± 13.8
10 min	94.2 ± 5.0	91.7 ± 7.0	86.6 ± 10.9
20 min	97.4 ± 3.9	90.2 ± 8.9	98.8 ± 4.4

* Dorsum of the foot, skin temperature 29.5 ± 0.5°C elevated by an electric pad or decreased by a cold-hot pack (3M). ** Medial ankle, skin temperature 31.0 ± 0.5°C
In the first study (1), the area of densitometric measurement was 2 mm^2, in the second (30) 2.8 mm^2, and in the third (23) 3.2 mm^2.

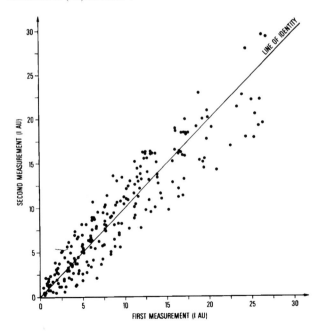

Figure 46. Reproducibility of individual fluorescent light intensity values measured in arbitrary units (AU). The skin area of 2 mm^2 covered by the large window densitometer was located at the dorsum of the foot. The measurements were performed at day 1 ("first measurement") and 2 days later ("second measurement") with a controlled skin temperature of 29.5 ± 0.5°C. The correlation coefficient was r = 0.84.

Single capillary studies have the advantage of optimal spatial resolution permitting determination of fluorescent light intensity in selected sections of the interstitial space. On the other hand, measurements of fluorescent light intensity in larger *skin areas* with a relatively small magnification (see page page 42) yield more representative values for a group of microvessels.

The mean values of three studies are plotted in **Table 10**, obtained at the dorsum of the foot and at the medial ankle, respectively. After the first study (1) a new brand of NaF had to be used (23, 30) because the old dye was no longer available. In vitro testing revealed that FLI emanating from the second 20% NaF solution reached only about 60% the intensity emanating from the previously used dye. Each laboratory should establish its own normal values and consider that control and patient groups have to be examined by identical procedures and identical dye brands.

Test-retest experiments in the same healthy volunteers using identical dye and procedure revealed a satisfactory reproducibility at the foot dorsum, provided that skin temperature was kept at 29.5 ± 0.5°C (1). The correlation coefficient between the values measured at day one and three was r = 0.84 (**Figure 46**; 1). When skin temperature was not standardized, reproducibility was not satisfactory.

References 1.3

1) Baer-Suryadinata, Ch., Bollinger, A.: Transcapillary diffusion of Na-fluorescein measured by a "large window technique" in skin areas of the forefoot. *Int. J. Microcirc.: Clin. Exp.* 4, 217–228, 1985.
2) Bollinger, A., Jäger, K., Roten, A., Timeus, Ch., Mahler, F.: Diffusion, pericapillary distribution and clearance of Na-fluorescein in the human nailfold. *Pflügers Arch.* 382, 137–143, 1979.
3) Bollinger, A., Jäger, K., Sgier, F., Seglias, J.: Fluorescence microlymphography. *Circulation* 64, 1195–1200, 1981.
4) Bollinger, A., Frey, J., Jäger, K., Furrer, J., Siegenthaler, W.: Patterns of diffusion through skin capillaries in patients with long-term diabetes. *New Engl. J. Med.* 307, 1305–1310, 1982.
5) Bollinger, A., Partsch, H., Wolfe, J. H. N. (eds.): *The initial lymphatics, new methods and findings.* Thieme, Stuttgart, New York, 1985.
6) Bollinger, A., Jünger, M., Jäger, K.: Fluorescence video microscopy techniques for the evaluation of human skin microcirculation. *Prog. appl. Microcirc.* 11, 77–97, 1986.
7) Brülisauer, M., Bollinger, A.: Measurement of different human microvascular dimensions by combination of video microscopy with Na-fluorescein (NaF) and indocyanine green (ICG) in normals and patients with systemic sclerosis. *Int. J. Microcirc.: Clin. Exp.* (in print).
8) Burcynski, F. J., Greenway, C. V., Sitar, D. S.: Hepatic blood flow: Accuracy of estimation from infusions of indocyanine green in anaesthetized cats. *Br. J. Pharmac.* 91, 651–659, 1987.
9) Carski, T. R., Staller, B. J., Hepner, G., Banka, V. S., Finney, R. A.: Adverse reactions after administration of indocyanine green. *J. Am. Med. Ass.* 240, 635, 1978.
10) Chen, P. C. Y., Kovalcheck, S. W., Zweifach, B. W.: Analysis of microvascular network in bulbar conjunctiva by image processing. *Int. J. Microcirc.: Clin. Exp.* 6, 245–255, 1987.
11) Dagher, F. J., Lyons, J. H., Finlayson, D. C., Shamsai, J., Moore, F. D.: Blood volume measurement: A critical study prediction of normal values: Controlled measurement of sequential changes. *Adv. Surg.* 1, 69–109, 1965.
12) Enzmann, V., Ruprecht, K. W.: Zwischenfälle bei der Fluoreszenzangiographie der Retina. Symptomatik, Prophylaxe und Therapie. *Klin. Mbl. Augenheilk.* 181, 235–239, 1982.
13) Fåhraeus, R., Lindqvist, T.: The viscosity of the blood in narrow capillary tubes. *Am. J. Physiol.* 96, 562–568, 1931.
14) Flower, R. W., Hochheimer, B. F.: A clinical technique and apparatus for simultaneous

angiography of the separate retinal and choroidal circulations. *Invest. Ophthalm.* 12, 248–261, 1973.

15) Flower, R. W., Hochheimer, B. F.: Indocyanine green dye fluorescence and infrared absorption choroidal angiography performed simultaneously with fluorescein angiography. *John Hopkins Med. J.* 138, 33–142, 1976.

16) Fox, I. J., Wood, E. H.: Applications of dilution curves recorded from the right side of the heart or venous circulation with the aid of a new indicator dye. *Proc. Staff Meet. Mayo Clinic* 32, 541–550, 1957.

17) Fox, I. J., Wood, E. H.: Indocyanine green: Physical and physiologic properties. *Proc. Staff Meet. Mayo Clinic* 35, 732–744, 1960.

18) Franzeck, U. K., Isenring, G., Frey, J., Jäger, K., Mahler, F., Bollinger, A.: Eine Apparatur zur dynamischen intravitalen Videomikroskopie. *VASA* 12, 233–238, 1983.

19) Franzeck, U. K., Isenring, G., Frey, J., Bollinger, A.: Videodensitometric pattern recognition of Na-fluorescein diffusion in nailfold capillary areas of patients with acrocyanosis, primary vasospastic and secondary Raynaud's phenomenon. *Inter. Angiol.* 2, 143–152, 1983.

20) Frey, J., Furrer, J., Bollinger, A.: Transkapillare Diffusion von Na-Fluoreszein in Hautarealen des Fußrückens bei juvenilen Diabetikern. *Schweiz. med. Wschr.* 113, 1964–1969, 1983.

21) Gaehtgens, P.: "Regulation" of capillary haematocrit. *Int. J. Microcirc.: Clin. Exp.* 3, 147–160, 1984.

22) Grassi, W., Gasparini, M., Adamo, V., Pietropaolo, N., Cervini, C.: L'analisi morfometrica computerizzata nello studio delle microangiopatie: Recenti progressi. *Acta Cardiol. Medit.* 3, 129–136, 1985.

23) Haselbach, P., Vollenweider, U., Moneta, G., Bollinger, A.: Microangiopathy of severe chronic venous insufficiency evaluated by fluorescence video microscopy. *Phlebology* 1, 159–169, 1986.

24) Higgins, J. C., Eady, R. A. J.: Human dermal microvasculature: I. Its segmental differentiation. Light and electron microscopic study. *Br. J. Dermatol.* 104, 117–129, 1981.

25) Hunton, D. B., Bollmann, J. L., Hoffmann, H. N.: Studies on hepatic function with indocyanine green. *Gastroenterology* 39, 713–724, 1960.

26) Intaglietta, M., Johnson, P. C.: Principle of capillary exchange. In Johnson P. C. (ed.): *Peripheral circulation.* John Wiley and Sons, New York, Chichester, Brisbane, Toronto. pp. 141–166, 1978.

27) Intaglietta, M., Tompkins, W. R.: Contrast enhancement amplifier for television microscopy. *Int. J. Microcir.: Clin. Exp.* 7, 253–260, 1988.

28) Jacobs, M. J. H. M., Breslau, P. J., Slaaf, D. W., Reneman, R. S., Lemmens, J. A. J.: Nomenclature of Raynaud's phenomenon: A capillary microsopic and hemorheologic study. *Surgery* 101, 136–145, 1987.

29) Jäger, K., Geser, A., Bollinger, A.: Videodensitometrische Messung der transkapillaren Passage und Gewebsverteilung von Na-Fluorezein in menschlichen Hautkapillaren. *VASA* 9, 132–136, 1980.

30) Jünger, M., Frey-Schnewlin, G., Bollinger, A.: Microvascular flow distribution and transcapillary diffusion at the forefoot in patients with peripheral ischemia. *Int. J. Microcirc.: Clin. Exp.* 8, 3–24, 1989.

31) Kjaergaard, J. J., Dideriksen, K., Mourits-Anderson, T.: Some aspects of the pharmacokinetics of fluorescein in normals and in diabetic subjects. *Int. J. Microcirc.: Clin. Exp.* 2, 191–197, 1983.

32) Kjaergaard, J. J., Fabrin, K.: Some methodological problems in ocular fluorophotometry. *Int. J. Microcirc.: Clin. Exp.* 2, 177–189, 1983.

33) Kogure, K., Choromokes, E.: Infrared absorption angiography. *J. Appl. Physiol.* 26, 154–157, 1969.

34) Ley, K., Pries, A. R., Gaehtgens, P.: A versatile intravital microscope design. *Int. J. Microcirc.: Clin. Exp.* 6, 161–167, 1987.

35) Lund, F.: Fluorescein angiography, an overview of technical improvements and recent experiences in previous and new clinical areas of application. *Biblthca. anat.* 18, 322–327, 1979.

36) Mahler, F., Nagel, G., Saner, H., Kneubühl, F.: In vivo comparison of the nailfold capil-

lary diameter as determined by using the erythrocyte column and FITC-albumin. *Int. J. Microcirc.: Clin. Exp.* 2, 147–155, 1983.

37) Meijer, E. K. F., Weert, B., Vermeer, G. A.: Pharmacokinetics of biliary excretion in man. VI. Indocyanine Green. *Eur. J. Pharmacol.* 35, 295–303, 1985.

38) Moneta, G., Brülisauer, M., Jäger, K., Bollinger, A.: Infrared fluorescence video microscopy of skin capillaries with indocyanine green. *Int. J. Microcirc.: Clin. Exp.* 6, 25–34, 1987.

39) Muckle, T. J.: Plasma protein binding of indocyanine green. *Biochem. Med.* 15, 17–21, 1976.

40) Oedland, G. F.: The fine structure of cutaneous capillaries. In E. W. Montagna, R. A. Ellis (eds.), *Advances in biology of skin*. Pergamon Press, New York 2, 57–70, 1961.

41) Perbeck, L., Lund, F., Svensson, L., Thulin, L.: Fluorescein flowmetry: A method for measuring relative capillary blood flow in the intestine. *Clin. Physiol.* 5, 281–292, 1985.

42) Pilger, E.: Computergestützte In-vivo-Untersuchung der Kapillarpermeabilität. *Wien. Med. Wschr. Suppl.* 94, 2–42, 1985.

43) Pries, A. R.: A versatile video image analysis system for microcirculatory research. *Int. J. Microcirc.: Clin. Exp.* 7, 327–345, 1988.

44) Reed, M. W. R., Miller, F. N.: Importance of light dose in fluorescent microscopy. *Microvasc. Res.* 36, 104–197, 1988.

45) Saner, H., Boss, Ch., Mahler, F.: Demonstration of the pericapillary space after intravenous administration of sodium fluorescein. In A. Bollinger, H. Partsch, J. H. N. Wolfe (eds.). *The initial lymphatics*. Thieme, Stuttgart, New York, 94–97, 1985.

46) Slaaf, D. W., Tangelder, G. J., Reneman, R. S., Jäger, K., Bollinger, A.: A versatile incident illuminator for intravital microscopy. *Int. J. Microcirc.: Clin. Exp.* 6, 391–397, 1987.

47) Waldhausen, E., Marquardt, E., Helms, U.: Erfahrungen aus 31 anaphylaktoiden Reaktionen. *Anaesthesist* 30, 47–51, 1981.

48) Wayland, H., Hock, J.: Application of fluorescence vital microscopy to the vasculature around erupting teeth. *Microvasc. Res.* 7, 201–206, 1974.

49) Wessing, A.: *Fluoreszenzangiographie der Retina*. Thieme, Stuttgart, 1968.

50) Wheeler, H. O., Cranston, W. I., Meltzer, J. I.: Hepatic uptake and biliary excretion of indocyanine green in the dog. *Proc. Soc. Exp. Biol. Med.* 99, 11–14, 1958.

1.4 Fluorescence Microlymphography

Unlike blood capillaries microlymphatics are not visualized by conventional capillaroscopy or by fluorescence video microscopy using NaF or ICG as tracers. However, they may be stained by macromolecular fluorescent materials (FITC-dextran 150,000, FITC-human albumin), which are injected into the subepidermal layer of any part of the skin (2, 9). From the original interstitial deposit, the dye moves into the superficial network of lymphatic microvessels and renders them visible. The large molecules are almost exclusively drained by the lymphatic system. The capillaries are depicted by an incident light fluorescent microscope identical to the one used for NaF studies.

Patent blue injected for visualization of larger vessels (conventional lymphography) is not suited to coloring microvessels (2). It spreads into the superficial tissue diffusely, probably because of its low molecular weight. On the other hand, it can be used diagnosticly for depicting macrovessels from a subepidermal depot.

Anatomy of Skin Microlymphatics

Textbooks of anatomy still do not contain much information about small lymphatic vessels. Kubik (12) has shown that the microlymphatics of the skin form two superficial networks interconnected by channels running perpendicular to the surface (**Figure 47**). Both networks are composed of regular meshes arranged parallel to the skin surface. Several blood capillary loops that emerge from below are encircled by one mesh. Still deeper than the second superficial network, precollectors drain the fluid toward the large trunks. The latter empty into the first lymph nodes interposed into lymphatic transport to the large intraabdominal and intrathoracic ducts.

The density of network meshes is highest at the extremities, such as at the big toe, and be-

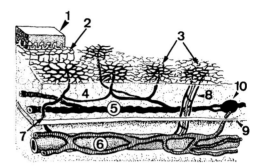

Figure 47. Schematic anatomical drawing of skin lymphatic microvessels according to Kubik (12). Two networks of initial lymphatics (lymphatic capillaries) are superposed (2 and 3) and connected by channels running perpendicular to the skin surface (4). There are also connecting vessels (7 and 8) to deeper subfascial lymphatics (6). Precollectors (5) drain the fluid from the deeper network toward the collectors (10).

comes lower in more proximal parts like at the ankle region (2, 9, 12). The diameter of microlymphatics is considerably larger than that of blood capillaries. Values determined in vivo are given below.

Like blood capillaries, lymphatic microvessels are lined by thin endothelial cells. Whereas the endothelial cell lining is continuous, the surrounding basal laminae are often indistinct and discontinuous (4, 5). Anchoring filaments (4, 13) are attached to the cells, and they are stretched when interstitial pressure is elevated. By this mechanism the interendothelial clefts are widely opened in order to enhance fluid flow from the interstitial space into the initial lymphatics. With low interstitial volume and pressure, the filaments are loose and the clefts closed or only slightly open.

Before fluid and macromolecules enter the lymphatic capillaries, they move in the interstitial space on preferential prelymphatic pathways. Among the latter, elastic fibers are of particular importance (6). In humans, there is some evidence that prelymphatic channels run close to the skin blood capillary loops (see page 103 and **Figure 77**).

Dyes

FITC-dextran with a molecular weight of 150,000 has been widely used as an intravital fluorescent dye for staining skin lymphatic microvessels (2, 3, 8, 9, 16). FITC (**fluorescein isothiocyanate**) coupled to the dextran molecule renders the compound visible below the fluorescence microscope. The substance is available in powder form (Sigma) and is dissolved in physiologic saline solution under sterile conditions to form a 25% solution of the macromolecular dye.

When injected subepidermally in minute amounts not much superior to a mosquito sting, FITC-dextran 150,000 is well tolerated. More than 2,000 examinations have been performed so far without major side effects. Rarely, the dye provokes a harmless itching reaction. It should be kept in mind that the substance has not been subjected to tests allowing its intravenous use in humans.

In principle, other molecular sizes as well may be used for fluorescence microlymphography. As has been shown, FITC-dextran 40,000 also depicts microlymphatics, but in part returns to the interstitial space through the capillary wall (7).

In addition, FITC-labeled human albumin is appropriate for coloring lymphatic capillaries (14). It cannot be purchased commercially. How FITC is coupled to human albumin, is described elsewhere (14).

Technique

The patient rests comfortably in a supine position. The most common examination site is the medial ankle region (2, 3, 8, 9, 16). The patient lies on his lateral side with the leg bent slightly ("shock position").

The investigation of the upper limb is usually performed on the palmar aspect of the lower arm (1). Other sites of injection like the face, abdomen, or thigh have been used occasionally.

Identical fluorescence microscopes and filters as described for the application of the dye NaF (see page 35) are suited for microlymphography. For an overview of the dye depot and the field of depicted microlymphatics, objectives with small magnification are preferred. An adequate objective is the plan 1/0.04 with a final magnification of 36× on a small television screen. Larger magnifications are used for documenting details of microvascular anatomy or for measuring permeability of lymphatic capillaries.

A microneedle and a microsyringe are used (**Figure 48**) for injecting 0.005–0.05 ml of a 25% solution of FITC-dextran 150,000. The dosage applied in most instances is 0.01 ml. Larger amounts create depots of undesirably large dimensions. The steel cannula (Hamilton) has an external diameter of 0.2 mm and is incorporated into a needle holder. The microsyringe (Hamilton, Mohler) has a total volume of 50 µl so that one unit corresponds to 1 µl. The small dimension of the needle and the minute volume injected guarantee that the puncture causes only minimal discomfort to the patient and minor alteration of the physiologic situation.

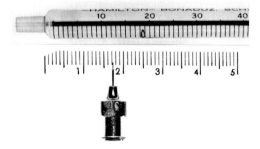

Figure 48. Microneedle and microsyringe (Hamilton) used for fluorescence microlymphography. The top of the steel cannula (Hamilton) melted into a large cylinder has an outer diameter of 0.2 mm.

Fluorescence Microlymphography

Since it is difficult to fill the microsyringe and cannula directly, the indicator substance is drawn from the ampoule into an insulin syringe (1 ml) and then injected into microsyringe and steel cannula. The viscous substance dries quickly and should be made ready for use just prior to injection.

After having disinfected the skin surface, place the tip of the cannula subepidermally at an acute angle to the skin and inject the dye as gently as possible. A brightly fluorescing spot, easily recognized below the fluorescence microscope (**Figure 49**), is created. If the deposit is not clearly visualized, an inadequately deep injection site should be suspected, and the procedure should be repeated at another location nearby. Deposits placed into a deeper skin layer may fail to stain the lymphatic capillaries. The application of several dye depots in the region of interest is recommended.

While manual injection is adequate for routine microlymphography, the use of a micromanipulator is advisable for special scientific purposes. It allows precise placing of the dye deposit under microscopic control.

The network of lymphatic capillaries is filled from the dye depot in the interstitial space (**Figure 49**). For the most part, the microvessels fill immediately after the end of injection or within the first minutes. A drop of paraffin oil on the skin optimizes image quality.

The dynamics of dye spread into the network of microlymphatics are observed for 20–60 minutes by the video microscopy system described for application of NaF. Documentation is performed either by periodic tape recordings or by photography with a high-speed fluorescence sensitive film (Kodak). Photographs may also be taken of single frames of the television recordings displayed on the monitor.

Evaluation and Normal Findings

The evaluation of the images obtained includes description of morphological and functional parameters (intact network, obliterations, early blurring because of increased permeability),

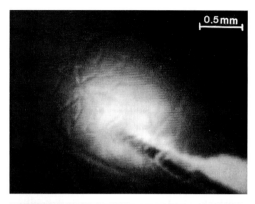

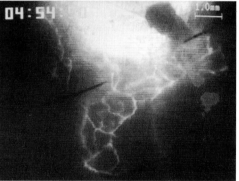

Figure 49.
Above: Microneedle inserted into the subepidermal layer below the fluorescence microscope. The depot of FITC-dextran 150,000 has just been placed and appears as a bright spot.
Below: 4 min and 54 s after FITC-dextran 150,000 injection. The depot is visualized in the upper part of the image. Some meshes of lymphatic capillaries have been stained by the macromolecular fluorescent dye in the lower part.

measurements of capillary diameters, and of dye spread into the network.

The superficial lymphatic capillaries filled from the deposit of FITC-dextran 150,000 form a regular *network* composed of more or less tight meshes. The second deeper network located in the subcutis is not visualized. In about one-third of normal controls, the superficial part of connecting vessels plunging toward the deeper layers is identified (8).

The *physiologic extension* of the macromolecular dye into the network is limited to one or a few meshes (**Figure 49**). In most instances, less than 20 meshes are visualized (8). This is probably because lymphatic flow into deeper channels is not impeded in normals. The fluorescent macromolecules are transported into the large vessels without depiction of an extended superficial capillary network.

The extension of the depicted network from the edge of the dye deposit is measured on the television screen at low magnification. The border of the depot is relatively well defined, as are the most distant microvessels depicted. The measurements are performed when dye filling has reached its maximal extension. Usually, the filling of the network lasts no more than 10–15 minutes.

Normal values of dye spread into the four directions were determined at the medial ankle (8); these are given in **Table 11**. It is recommended to measure the extension of the depicted network into the proximal, distal, ventral, and dorsal part of the depicted network. In addition, the maximal extension into one of the four directions is noted. The upper normal value for maximal spread at the ankle region is 12 mm (8). Increased spread of the dye is diagnosed when maximal extension exceeds this limit.

Table 11. Mean spread of FITC-dextran 150,000 in superficial lymphatic capillaries of the medial ankle measured in mm from the outer limit of the dye deposit (Isenring et al., 8).

Direction	Extension
Proximal	3.5 ± 2.5
Distal	2.9 ± 2.1
Ventral	3.9 ± 2.9
Dorsal	7.1 ± 3.2
Maximal (in any direction)	7.8 ± 2.6

When the microinjection is performed close to the nailfold of the big toe, a network composed of dense meshes is visualized (2, 9) that extends on the dorso-lateral aspect of the toe (see **Figure 84**, page 110).

As will be shown later (page 110), increased parts of the network are stained in patients with lymphedema and phlebedema in whom flow into the hypoplastic or partially obliterated pre-collectors is reduced, intact superficial microlymphatics acting as a compensatory basin.

Measurements of lymphatic capillary diameters are useful especially in patients with congenital lymphedema (3, 16). Single frames of television recordings are displayed on the video screen, and the diameters of at least 10 initial lymphatics are measured by a caliper. The mean value calculated characterizes individual capillary width. The values are estimates, since the vessel edge is not precisely delineated. Some scattering of transmitted light cannot be avoided. Alternative methods for diameter measurements employ image-shearing monitors or image-analysis systems.

For scientific purposes, a raster may be attached to the monitor subdividing the image into a number of quadratic fields. Within each field the microvessel with optimal delineation and lowest light scattering is selected for diameter determination (16).

In healthy controls, the mean lymphatic capillary diameter at the ankle reached 56.3 ± 9.0 μm (medium 52.8 μm, range 45–73 μm; 16). In this investigation the morphometric technique described above was used. Earlier work with a less standardized technique of evaluation yielded a mean value of 81 ± 16.6 μm (8). The light scattering mentioned is probably the main reason for the varying results between different observers. When comparing normal values to values determined in patients, it is essential that identical trained observers evaluate both normal and pathologic findings.

Measurement of Lymphatic Capillary Permeability

Macromolecules are drained by the lymphatic system back into the veins. Under certain circumstances, they may move through the capillary wall and reenter the interstitial compartment (10). Therefore, permeability of initial lymphatics means return of macromolecules to the interstitial space by crossing endothelial

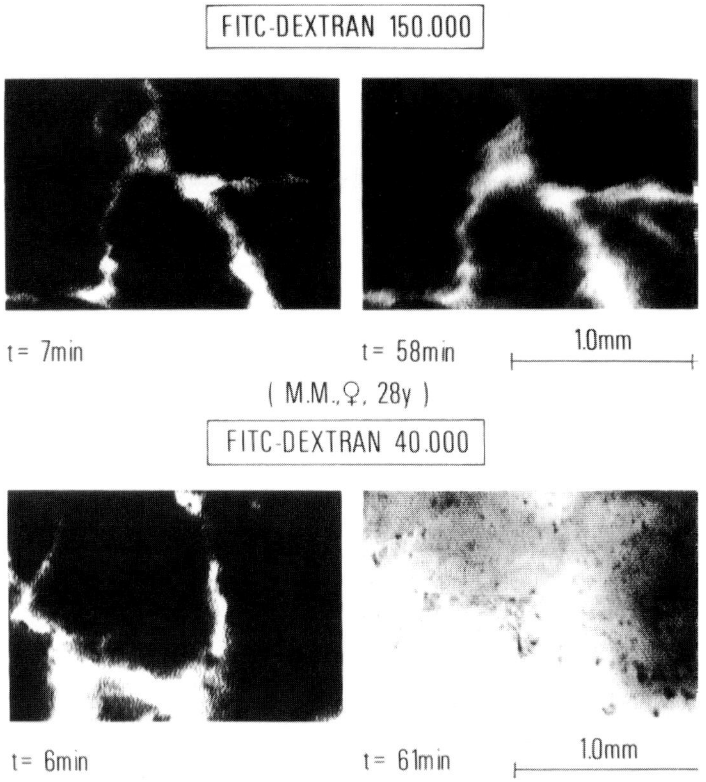

Fluorescence Microlymphography

FITC-DEXTRAN 150.000

t = 7min   t = 58min   1.0mm

(M.M., ♀, 28y)

FITC-DEXTRAN 40.000

t = 6min   t = 61min   1.0mm

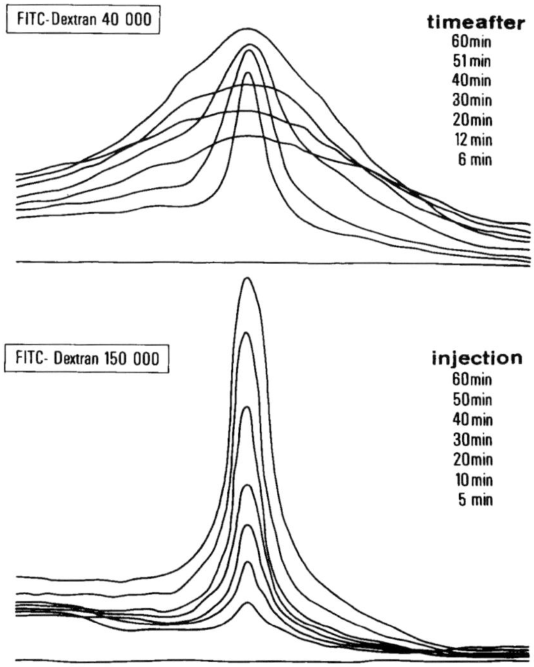

FITC-Dextran 40 000

time after
60 min
51 min
40 min
30 min
20 min
12 min
6 min

FITC-Dextran 150 000

injection
60 min
50 min
40 min
30 min
20 min
10 min
5 min

Figure 50.
Above (a): Mesh of initial lymphatics visualized by FITC-dextrans 150,000 and 40,000, respectively. The capillaries appear well delineated soon after dye injection, but about 1 hour later only through use of the larger molecule. Bright interstitial fluorescence is recorded with the smaller molecule 61 min after injection since the dye has leaked out of the capillary lumen.
Below (b): Fluorescent light intensities determined by video densitometry on an axis crossing a single lymphatic microvessel at various times. Slim peaks of intensity remain located over the capillary for 1 h with FITC-dextran 150,000. With the molecular weight of 40,000, the steep descending slopes of the tracings flatten and move away from the capillary wall.

cells and basal lamina or by passing interendothelial clefts.

The permeability of microlymphatics may be determined by video densitometry or image analysis like that described for transcapillary diffusion of NaF (7). In fact, molecules not only enter the initial lymphatics leaving the interstitial space, under certain conditions they may permeate through the wall and return to the interstitium.

Video recordings of identical network sections are obtained at different times and displayed as single frames on the television monitor. The densitometer line on which fluorescent light intensities are recorded crosses the lymphatic capillary at a right angle and at a defined site (**Figure 50a**).

In **Figure 50b**, representative tracings are plotted that were obtained in a healthy volunteer with two molecular sizes. Without permeation of the dye, high peaks of fluorescent light intensity remain located over the capillary (FITC-dextran 150,000). Steep slopes of decreasing intensity indicate the site of the capillary wall. However, the steep gradients level off if smaller fluorescent molecules (FITC-dextran 40,000) cross the wall of the microvessel.

In normals, FITC-dextran 150,000 does not leak out of the intravascular compartment for up to 1 h, whereas the smaller molecule (40,000) first enters the initial lymphatics, but later leaves them in part. The corresponding images show well-delineated capillaries without leakage but with bright interstitial fluorescence around the microvessels permeable to the macromolecule (**Figure 50b**). In future studies, intermittent light exposure should be preferred in order to avoid increases of permeability due to prolonged illumination.

For evaluation of permeability, the usual technique of fluorescence microlymphography has to be modified (7). A group of well-delineated vessels as far away as possible from the dye depot is repeatedly visualized. Images are recorded on video tape at regular intervals. Dye movement from the deposit has to be distinguished from increased permeability of the capillary wall (7). Sites of light intensity measurement close to the microlymphatics are typical for the amount of permeating molecules and sites far away from the vessel for dye concentrations stemming from the depot.

Studies with more than two molecular sizes have not been performed so far. In principle, it should be possible to determine the range of molecular sizes staying within the microlymphatics and of others passing through the capillary wall under physiologic and pathologic conditions.

References 1.4

1) Baer-Suryadinata, Ch., Clodius, L., Isenring, G., Bollinger, A.: Lymph capillaries in postmastectomy lymphedema. In Bollinger, A., Partsch, H., Wolfe, J. H. N. (eds.) : *The initial lymphatics, new methods and findings*. Thieme, Stuttgart, New York, 158–181, 1985.

2) Bollinger, A., Jäger, K., Sgier, F., Seglias, J.: Fluorescence microlymphography. *Circulation* 64, 1195–1200, 1981.

3) Bollinger, A., Partsch, H., Wolfe, J. H. N. (eds.): *The initial lymphatics, new methods and findings*. Thieme, Stuttgart, New York, 1985.

4) Castenholz, A. : The demonstration of lymphatics in casts and fixed tissue with the scanning electron microscope. In Bollinger, A., Partsch, H., Wolfe, J. H. N. (eds.): *The initial lymphatics, new methods and findings*. Thieme, Stuttgart, New York, 75–83, 1985.

5) Hammersen, F., Hammersen, E. : On the fine structure of lymphatic capillaries. In Bollinger, A., Partsch, H., Wolfe, J. H. N. (eds.) : *The initial lymphatics, new methods and findings*. Thieme, Stuttgart, New York, 58–65, 1985.

6) Hauck, G. : Prelymphatic pathways,. In Bollinger, A., Partsch, H., Wolfe, J. H. N. (eds.): *The initial lymphatics, new methods and findings*. Thieme, Stuttgart, New York, 50–57, 1985.

7) Huber, M., Franzeck, U. K., Bollinger, A.: Permeability of superficial lymphatic capillaries in human skin to FITC-labeled dex-

trans 40,000 and 150,000. *Int. J. Microc.: Clin. Exp.* 3, 59–69, 1984.

8) Isenring, G., Franzeck, U. K., Bollinger, A.: Fluoreszenz-Mikrolymphographie am medialen Malleolus bei Gesunden und Patienten mit primärem Lymphödem. *Schweiz. med. Wschr.* 112, 225–231, 1982.

9) Jäger, K., Sgier, F., Seglias, J., Bollinger, A.: Fluorescence microlymphography. *Biblthca. anat.* 20, 712–715, 1981.

10) Johansson, B. R.: Permeability of muscle capillaries to interstitially microinjected horseradish peroxidase. *Microvasc. Res.* 16, 340–353, 1978.

11) Kinmonth, J. B.: *The lymphatics, surgery, lymphography and diseases of the chyle and lymph systems.* E. Arnold, London, 1982.

12) Kubik, St.: Anatomie des Lymphgefäßsystems. In Frommhold, W., Gerhardt, P. (eds.): *Erkrankungen des Lymphsystems.* Thieme, Stuttgart, New York, 1–19, 1981.

13) Leak, L. V.: The structure of lymphatic capillaries in lymph formation. *Fed. Proc.* 35, 1863–1871, 1976.

14) Mahler, F., Boss, Ch., Saner, H.: Microlymphography with FITC human albumin. In Bollinger, A., Partsch, H., Wolfe, J. H. N. (eds.): *The initial lymphatics, new methods and findings.* Thieme, Stuttgart, New York, 106–109, 1985.

15) Partsch, H., Wenzel-Hora, B. I., Urbanek, A.: Differential diagnosis of lymphedema after indirect lymphography with Iotasul. *Lymphology* 16, 12–18, 1983.

16) Pfister, G., Saesseli, B., Hoffmann, U., Geiger, M., Bollinger, A.: Diameter of lymphatic skin capillaries in different forms of primary lymphedema. *Lymphology* (in print).

17) Wenzel-Hora, B. I., Kalbas, B., Siefert H. M., Arndt, J. O., Schlösser, H. W., Huth, F.: Iotasul, a water-soluble (non-oily) contrast medium for direct and indirect lymphography. Radiological and morphological investigations in dogs. *Lymphology* 14, 101–112, 1981.

1.5 Combination of Techniques

The introduction of transcutaneous measurements of oxygen tension (8) and of laser Doppler fluxmetry (7, 13) for the study of skin microcirculation suggested their combination with capillaroscopy, since the latter technique permits direct insights into morphology and function of the microvessels relevant for the two noninvasive investigations.

Transcutaneous oxygen tension at 43°C–45°C ($tcPo_2$) depends primarily on the flow in the superficial capillaries of the skin. Under normal circulatory conditions, it reflects systemic arterial oxygen tension; under ischemic conditions, the values characterize the degree of ischemia in the skin region examined. Decreased values have been observed distal of arterial occlusions of limb arteries (1, 4, 10, 16) and in microangiopathy from severe chronic venous insufficiency at the medial ankle (5, 11, 12).

In contrast to the values measured by probes heated to 43–45°C, which correspond to almost maximal vasodilatation, the values at 37°C ($ssPo_2$) are low. However, they react promptly to vasodilating stimuli like timed arterial occlusion (reactive hyperemia).

Laser Doppler instruments record flux in a skin section of about one mm^3 (13). The sample volume comprises nutritive capillaries and more deeply localized shunt vessels. As shown by comparative measurements, fluctuations in capillary velocity at the nailfold are not always synchronous with changes of the laser Doppler output (3).

Flux is defined by the product of the number of moving blood cells in the sample volume and their velocity. It is expressed in arbitrary units and considered a relative indicator of cutaneous blood flow.

Combination of Capillaroscopy and Measurements of $tcPo_2$

A window probe has been manufactured allowing combination of capillaroscopy and determi-

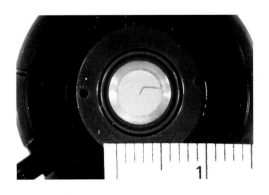 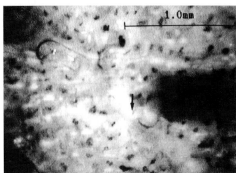

Figure 51. Combined probe for measurement of transcutaneous oxygen tension ($tcPO_2$) and capillaroscopy (from Franzeck et al., 5).
Left: Probe with transparent window through which capillaroscopy is performed. The platinum cathode for $tcPO_2$ measurements is melted into the glass cylinder. Its larger macroscopic part is easily recognized. *Right:* Capillaroscopic image at the medial ankle with capillaries appearing as dots or commas. The shadow on the right side corresponds to the distal part of the platinum cathode. The arrow indicates the small tip of the oxygen-sensing cathode. The location of the cathode may be precisely defined with respect to the underlying capillaries.

nation of $tcPo_2$ at identical sites (5, 9). **Figure 51** shows a prototype of the probe. The center is transparent and contains the platinum cathode melted into the glass cylinder. The cathode tapers off and has a tip diameter of only 15 µm. The tip is located near the surface of the probe adjacent to the skin. The silver/silver-chloride anode and the heating system are located in the probe ring encircling the transparent glass cylinder.

The probe is no more than 6 mm high in order to fit below a microscope objective with large working distance. The capillaries are observed through the transparent central part and the teflon membrane placed between probe and skin. The membrane is reasonably translucent and reduces image quality only to a minor degree.

After the probe is fixed on the skin by an adhesive ring, the platinum cathode is visualized through the microscope. The plane of focus is moved toward the skin surface until the small tip of the cathode becomes visible. The position of the tip is marked on the television monitor. Now, the plane of the capillary loops is focused. The marked position of the cathode may be correlated to microvessel anatomy underlying the $tcPo_2$ sensor. The $tcPo_2$ measured stems essentially from the microvessels observed near the cathode.

The distance between the cathode tip and the apex of the capillary loop is called *diffusion distance* (15) and corresponds to the distance the oxygen molecules have to travel from the intravascular compartment to the platinum cathode. The diffusion distance may be measured by intravital capillaroscopy. A digital length meter (Wild-Leitz), mounted on the microscope, records the distance during the process of focusing (15).

Direct correlation between cathode location and capillary morphology or density (5) has shown that there is a direct linear relationship between $tcPo_2$ and capillary density in patients with chronic venous incompetence (see page 101).

Combination of Capillaroscopy, $tcPo_2$ Measurements, and Laser Doppler Flux

A probe combining determinations of $tcPo_2$ and laser Doppler flux has been used in first studies (2, 6). A still more sophisticated probe was developed in our laboratory in cooperation with A. and R. Huch which permits correlation of the output of the laser Doppler and $tcPo_2$ instrument to the capillaroscopic image in identical skin areas. The laser Doppler sensor reaches the skin surface through a hole in the heatable anode ring of the system for measuring $tcPo_2$. Since the laser light with a wavelength of 632.8 nm disturbs the video image, a special filter (Balzers) is required to eliminate light components in the nanometer range of the laser probe and improve the quality of the video images.

First applications of the triple probe document its proper function. Simultaneous measurements during reactive hyperemia after arterial occlusion were performed. Reactive hyperemia was recorded by both laser Doppler and $tcPo_2$ probe. Simultaneously, NaF injected during arterial occlusion was released by the sudden cuff deflation and transcapillary diffusion measured by the large window technique (page 42) near the peak value of hyperemia.

Interest of Combined Probes

At present, the different combination probes are mainly of scientific interest. The most promising is the triple probe, which is now being tested in larger series of controls and patients.

A broad application of the combined probes allows new insights into the complex microvascular dynamics. For example, it will become possible to analyze decreased microvascular reactivity and increased transcapillary diffusion in patients with diabetic microangiopathy at identical sites of measurement. The effect of different forms of fluxmotion (14) on $tcPo_2$ and capillary exchange is another topic for future studies.

References 1.5

1) Creutzig, A., Dau, D., Caspary, L., Alexander, K.: Transcutaneous oxygen pressure measured at two different electrode temperatures in healthy volunteers and patients with arterial occlusive disease. *Int. J. Microcirc.: Clin. Exp.* 5, 373–380, 1987.
2) Ewald, U., Huch, A., Huch, R., Rooth, G.: Skin reactive hyperemia recorded by a combined tcPo$_2$ and laser Doppler sensor. *Adv. exp. Med. Biol.* 220, 231–234, 1987.
3) Fagrell, B., Intaglietta, M., Tsai, A. G., Östergren, J.: Combination of laser Doppler flowmetry and capillary microscopy for evaluating the dynamics of skin microcirculation. In Mahler, F., Messmer, K., Hammersen, F. (eds.) *Techniques in clinical capillary microscopy*. Prog. appl. Microcirc. Karger, Basel, 11, 30–39, 1986.
4) Franzeck, U. K., Talke, P., Bernstein, E. F., Golbranson, F. L., Fronek, A.: Transcutaneous Po$_2$ measurements in health and peripheral arterial occlusive disease. *Surgery* 91, 156–163, 1982.
5) Franzeck, U. K., Bollinger, A., Huch, R., Huch, A.: Transcutaneous oxygen tension and capillary morphologic characteristics and density in patients with chronic venous incompetence. *Circulation* 70, 806–811, 1984.
6) Franzeck, U. K., Stengele, B., Panradl, U., Wahl, P., Tillmanns, H.: Cutaneous reactive hyperemia in short-term and long-term type I diabetes—Continuous monitoring by a combined laser Doppler and transcutaneous oxygen probe. *VASA* 19, 8–15, 1990.
7) Holloway, G. A., Watkins, D. W.: Laser Doppler measurement of cutaneous blood flow. *J. Invest. Dermatol.* 69, 306–309, 1977.
8) Huch, R., Huch, A., Luebbers, D. W.: *Transcutaneous Po$_2$*. Thieme-Stratton Inc., New York, 1981.
9) Huch, A., Franzeck, U. K., Huch, R., Bollinger, A.: A transparent transcutaneous oxygen electrode for simultaneous studies of skin capillary morphology, flow dynamics and oxygenation. *Int. J. Microcirc.: Clin. Exp.* 2, 103–108, 1983.
10) Karanfilian, R. G., Lynch, T. G., Zirul, V. T., Padberg, F. T., Jamil, Z., Hobson II, R. W.: The value of laser Doppler velocimetry and transcutaneous oxygen tension determination in predicting healing of ischemic forefoot ulcerations and amputations in diabetic and nondiabetic patients. *J. Vasc. Surg.* 4, 511–516, 1986.
11) Mannarino, E., Pasqualini, L., Maragoni, E., Sanchini, R., Regni, O., Innocente, S.: Chronic venous incompetence and transcutaneous oxygen pressure: A controlled study. *VASA* 17, 159–161, 1988.
12) Neumann, H. A. M., Leeuwen van, M., Broek van den, M. J. T. B., Berretty, P. J. M.: Transcutaneous oxygen tension in chronic venous insufficiency syndrome. *VASA* 13, 213–219, 1984.
13) Nilsson, G. E., Tenland, T., Oeberg, P. A.: Evaluation of a laser Doppler flowmeter for measurement of tissue blood flow. *IEEE Trans. Biomed. Eng.* 27, 597–604, 1980.
14) Seifert, H., Jäger, K., Bollinger, A.: Analysis of flow motion by the laser Doppler technique in patients with peripheral arterial occlusive disease. *Int. J. Microcirc.: Clin. Exp.* 7, 223–236, 1988.
15) Vesti, B., Franzeck, U. K., Geiger, M., Hoffmann, U., Bollinger, A.: Experimentelle Untersuchungen bei Bindegewebserkrankungen. *VASA*, Suppl. 27, 51–54, 1989.
16) White, R. A., Nolan, L., Harley, D., Long, J., Klein, S., Tremper, K., Nelson, R., Tabrisky, J., Shoemaker, W.: Noninvasive evaluation of peripheral vascular disease using transcutaneous oxygen tension. *Amer. J. Surg.* 144, 68–75, 1982.

2

PATHOLOGICAL CONDITIONS

2.1 Arterial Occlusive Disease (Ischemia)

The main symptoms in patients with peripheral arterial occlusive disease (PAOD) are *claudication, rest pain,* and *skin necrosis or gangrene.* All of these symptoms result from a reduction of the blood flow in the nutritional capillaries below the demand of that tissue for a certain moment. Studying the morphological pattern of the capillaries of the human muscle is presently not possible, but the nutritional skin capillaries can be easily studied by the described technique of vital capillaroscopy. In the late 1960s, preliminary observations of the capillaries of the dorsal skin of the foot and toes showed significant changes of nutritional skin capillaries in patients with PAOD (15). Extensive investigations later proved that capillaroscopy is one of the most sensitive methods for estimating the nutritional status of a certain skin area in patients with arteriosclerosis (9, 10). It has been shown that specific morphological changes of the nutritional capillaries appear with a successive decrease of the arterial circulation of the extremity. These changes can be classified and used for determining disturbances of the nutritional circulation in that particular skin area, and the risk of skin necrosis to develop can be accurately estimated (10, 11, 12, 14, 21).

Changes of Capillary Morphology

All skin areas of the body in which a diseased state is present can be investigated by ordinary capillaroscopy. However, the region most often studied is the skin of the foot. The reason for this is that the majority of patients with PAOD have their ischemic symptoms in the foot.

Investigating Procedure

In order to ensure good blood filling of the vascular bed under observation, the observed part of the extremity should be below heart level. This is of particular importance in patients with a markedly reduced arterial circulation, because when such an extremity is at, or above, heart level, no blood enters the ischemic region, and the vessels are empty of blood. When the foot and toes are studied, the patients should therefore be in a sitting position with the feet placed comfortably on a small table (see **Figure 4**, page 3). Paraffin oil is applied to the skin area before investigation, and the microscopic observation should start at a low magnification ($\approx 10\times$) to get a good overview over a larger area.

For technical and practical reasons, only the dorsal skin of the foot and toes is available for routine investigations in clinical practice. The normal pattern of the nutritional capillaries in this area is described on page 5.

Patients with PAOD

In patients with mild obliterative arteriosclerosis, the capillary bed of the forefoot does not seem to differ much from the normal pattern (10). Only patients with moderately or severly reduced arterial circulation to the area show any marked capillary alterations. In patients with only a minor decrease of the arterial circulation, the blood flow in the nutritional vascular bed is not reduced, so that no changes of the capillaries are present. A specific classification system has been used for documenting the morphological changes, and the following patterns can be observed in patients with PAOD:

Basic Classification

Normal stages (see also Chapter 1.1)

— Stage 0: Small dot- or comma-shaped capillaries. Good "tonicity" (**Figure 8 A**)
  This is the normal appearance of the capillaries of the foot and toes (see pages 5–7).

— Stage 1: Similar to Stage 0 but with less "tonicity" (**Figure 8 A**)
  The microvascular bed is more dilated, and in elderly subjects a few micropools may be seen (pages 5–7).

Pathological stages

— Stage 2: Dilatation of papillary capillaries (**Figure 8, A2**)
  A moderate or marked dilatation of the nutritional capillaries can be observed in most patients with PAOD. In several patients this dilatation appears as an aneurysm, which is classified as a "micropool" (arrows in **Figure 8**) (6, 11, 18). Sometimes these micropools can be 40–50 μm in diameter. The blood filling of the capillaries is also more uniform, and the normal tonicity seems to be lost.

— Stage 3: Indistinct capillaries (**Figure 8, B3 and 4**)
  In some patients with PAOD, the capillaries appear indistinct and cannot be sharply focused in the microscope. This most often is the result of edema formation or structural changes in the skin papillae themselves.

— Stage 4: Capillary haemorrhages (**Figure 8 B**)
  Extravasation of blood cells, indicating vast damage to the capillary wall, is seen in patients with severely reduced arterial circulation to the region. These changes are sometimes hard to distinguish from micropools, but the application of a light pressure to the structure in question shows that the micropools empty of blood by this procedure and become invisible, while the haemorrhages do not.

— Stage 5: Reduced number of blood filled capillaries (**Figure 8 C**)
  In prenecrotic states, there is a marked reduction in the number of visible, blood-filled capillaries in the area.

— Stage 6: No visible capillaries (**Figure 8 C**)
  Even though the patients are in the sitting position during the investigation, the capillaries can sometimes be completely empty of blood. This means that the blood does not reach the nutritional capillaries of the skin, and the risk of necrosis in these areas is imminent.

Comments: The presented classification with seven different stages has been shown to be unnecessarily sophisticated, and sometimes it can be difficult to differentiate them, for example, between Stage 0 and 1, which from the clinical point of view is of no practical importance. A simplified classification system was therefore introduced by Fagrell and Lundberg in 1984 (14), which has been shown to be very sensitive for evaluating the viability of the skin in patients with ischemia.

Simplified Classificaton System of Skin Capillaries

In this system, the different stages of the more sophisticated classification system described above are grouped together according to the following principle (**Figure 8**):

— Stages 0–2 = Stage A.

— Stages 3–4 = Stage B

— Stages 5–6 = Stage C

Relation Between Digital Arterial Circulation and Capillary Stage

The correlation between the arterial circulation of a certain digit, as evaluated by the systolic blood pressure (SBP) of the digit, and the capillary stages of the same digit, has been extensively studied; one example of this relationship is shown in **Figure 52**.

In toes with a SBP of more than 90 mmHg, the capillaries are usually normal (Stages 0 and 1). Also in toes with a SBP of 30 to 89 mmHg, the capillaries are normal or only slightly changed (Stage 0 to 2). Capillary haemorrhages (Stage 4) or edema (Stage 3) are seen in only 4–5%. In toes with a SBP of less than 30 mmHg, the whole spectrum of capillary morphology can be seen. Severe changes (Stages 5 and 6) are almost exclusively seen in toes with a high risk of, or already present, skin ulcers.

The simplified system was used in 122 patients with severe PAOD to test its value for predicting the risk of skin necrosis developing in the area (14). The patients, who all had a SBP value of the foot of 30 mmHg or less, were separated into three groups: 0–10, 11–20, 21–30 mmHg. The morphological changes of the capillaries were classified as Stage A, B, or C, and the patients were then clinically followed for at least 3 months, to record whether the patients developed a skin necrosis or gangrene

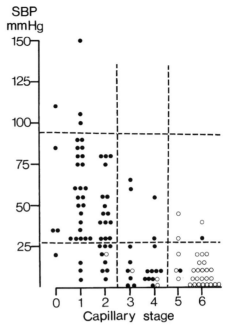

Figure 52. The relationship between capillary stage and systolic blood pressure of the big toe (SBP). At higher SBP (>90 mmHg) only normal capillaries can be seen. At very low pressures (<30 mmHg), the whole spectrum of capillary morphologies can be observed, but those patients who developed skin necrosis (o) had almost exclusively marked structural changes of the nutritional capillaries. All those where no skin necrosis developed (•) had blood-filled capillaries, although some of them were destroyed with edema and capillary hemorrhages.

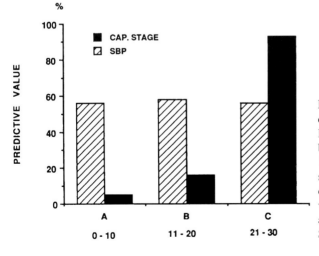

Figure 53. The predictive value for the development of skin necrosis of capillary stages (A, B, and C) and systolic blood pressure of the big toe (SBP 0–10, 11–20, 21–30 mmHg). It can be seen that stage C has a very high predictive value (96%) for the risk of developing skin necrosis in an area over an observation period of 3 months. SBP reached only 58%.

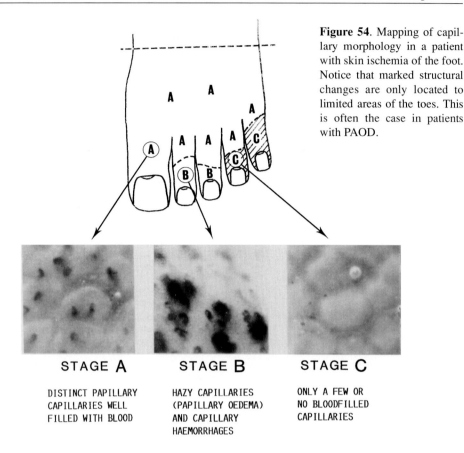

Figure 54. Mapping of capillary morphology in a patient with skin ischemia of the foot. Notice that marked structural changes are only located to limited areas of the toes. This is often the case in patients with PAOD.

STAGE A
DISTINCT PAPILLARY
CAPILLARIES WELL
FILLED WITH BLOOD

STAGE B
HAZY CAPILLARIES
(PAPILLARY OEDEMA)
AND CAPILLARY
HAEMORRHAGES

STAGE C
ONLY A FEW OR
NO BLOODFILLED
CAPILLARIES

in the investigated foot. The predictive values for the development of ulcers for Stage A, B, and C were 5%, 16%, and 93%, respectively (**Figure 53**).

Also, the specificity and sensitivity were tested. If the borderline was between Stage A and B+C, the sensitivity was 97% and the specificity 53%; put between Stage A+B and C, it was 87% and 95%, respectively. Consequently, the change in capillary structure was found to be a much more sensitive indicator for predicting the development of skin necrosis than the SBP of the toes, which reached a maximal specificity of only 53% for any of the three groups.

Comments: It must be stressed that ischemic skin necrosis most often appears in localized areas, like one toe or over a bony prominence (4, 10). This is a strong reason why methods that can only measure the total circulation in a whole region, or that only give spot-like information of the microcirculation, cannot evaluate the risk of necrosis in a certain area. For technical reasons blood pressure measurements, for example, can only be performed in one or two toes. An evaluation of the circulation of other digits is consequently not possible. With capillaroscopy the "target organ" of ischemia, i.e., the nutritional skin capillaries, can be directly visualized *in the whole area susceptible to necrosis*, and a disturbed nutritional circulation of a limited region is easily detected in the microscope. An example of how this "capillary mapping" can be performed is shown in **Figure 54**.

Changes of Capillary Blood Cell Velocity (CBV)

Not only the morphology changes in patients with a reduced arterial circulation, but also the capillary blood flow is affected. These disturbances have been studied in both the fingers and toes of patients with PAOD.

PAOD of the Arm

Nailfold CBV has been studied at rest and during post occlusive hyperemia after a 1-minute arterial occlusion in patients with arterial obliterative disease in one arm (32). As seen in Table 12, the rCBV in nailfold capillaries was the same in the affected and the unaffected arm. The peak CBV (pCBV) during reactive hyperemia after 1-minute arterial occlusion also showed the same value in both arms, but there was a significant ($p<0.01$) prolongation of the time to pCBV. This indicates a disturbed regulatory function of the precapillary vascular bed in the low-pressure area, which is probably the explanation for the observed long time to pCBV. Similiar results have been achieved in cat muscle capillaries, where it was found that the time to pCBV was significantly prolonged at low arterial blood pressure (22).

PAOD of the Leg

Clinical observations in patients with PAOD of the leg indicate a discrepancy between the total and the nutritional skin microcirculation of the feet in these patients, suggesting a maldistribution of the local blood flow. In a recent study (3), the total skin microcirculation was evaluated by laser Doppler fluxmetry (LDF), and the blood flow in the nutritional skin capillaries (CBV) by dynamic capillaroscopy. This combination was simultaneously used to study the nailfold microcirculation in the big toe of 12 legs with various degrees of PAOD, using 10 legs of healthy subjects as controls. CBV was evaluated by the cross-correlation technique, using the CapiFlow® computerized program.

The nutritional blood flow (CBV) was similar in patients and controls, whereas the total

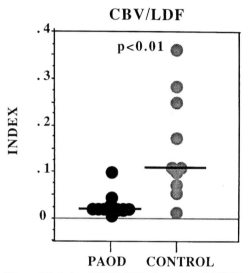

Figure 55. Index (CBV/LDF) of nutritional (CBV) versus nonnutritional (LDF) skin microcirculation in patients with peripheral arterial occlusive disease (PAOD) and controls. Median values are indicated by the horizontal bars.

Table 12. Reactivity of capillary blood cell velocity in 8 patients with PAOD of one arm. Values for the contralateral healthy arm are used as control ($\bar{x}\pm SD$).

	Arm with art. occl.	p value	Control arm
Finger BP (mmHg)	86 ± 14	<0.001	148 ± 20
Skin temp (°C)	28.1 ± 3.7	ns	28.9 ± 3.4
rCBV (mm/s)	0.39 ± 0.23	ns	0.48 ± 0.46
pCBV (mm/s)	0.57 ± 0.34	ns	0.69 ± 0.42
tpCBV (s)	20.0 ± 7.4	<0.01	11.6 ± 4.2

skin blood cell flux (LDF) in the same area was significantly *increased* in the patients in comparison to the normal subjects. However, the postocclusive reactive hyperemia response was impaired for both CBV and LDF in the PAOD group. The skin temperature was also significantly *higher* in the patients.

In order to get a rough estimation of how much blood reached the nutritional capillaries in the ischemic areas, the ratio between rCBV and rLDF was calculated (**Figure 55**). It was found that there was a marked decrease of this ratio in patients with PAOD as compared to controls. This indicates that there is a maldistribution of blood between nonnutritional and nutritional skin vessels of ischemic areas. The explanation for this is most probably that the ischemia triggers a dilatation of the arterioles and arteriovenous (AV) anastomoses of the nonnutritional, subpapillary vascular bed of the skin. The opening of the AV shunts gives rise to an increase of the pressure also in the venous system, keeping the AV pressure difference rather constant in the parallel coupled nutritional capillaries, which explains how the CBV can be unchanged or even decreased while the total skin blood flow is increased.

Comments: In spite of a significantly higher skin temperature and total skin blood flow in the PAOD patients, the capillary blood flow was not increased, indicating maldistribution of blood between nutritional and nonnutritional skin vessels. This increase in the total skin microcirculation in toes of PAOD patients is in full agreement with the results of McEvans and Ledingham (28). By using strain gauge pletysmography, they reported a significantly higher resting skin blood flow in clinically ischemic feet as compared to normals, but unfortunately they did not study the nutritional skin circulation in the region. Similar discrepancies between macro- and microcirculation have also been described by others (30).

Schwartz et al. (36) have also studied the CBV in toes of patients with PAOD, but they did not define the degree of arterial insufficiency in the investigated legs. They also studied the subjects in a sitting position, which sometimes influences the microcirculation rather dramatically because of the veni-vasomotor reflex that is triggered in the sitting position and leads to reduced skin circulation. They showed that the resting CBV was somewhat higher (n.s.) in the patients (0.16 mm/s) than in an elderly control group (0.10 mm/s), and a calculated capillary *flow* value (picoliters/s/mm^2) was also significantly (p<0.01) increased in the patients (281 pl/s/mm^2) as compared to the controls (85 pl/s/mm^2). These findings do not completely agree with the results of Bongard and Fagrell, perhaps because of the difference in the position during the investigation. Especially in patients with a marked reduction of the arterial inflow to a region is the arterial blood pressure much higher in the sitting than in the supine position, so that the results of the two studies cannot be compared. However, in both studies there was an impaired postocclusive hyperemia in the patients, which shows that the reactivity of the microvascular bed in patients with PAOD is more or less eliminated and may be less influenced by the position.

Flow-Motion Activity

Via the video-photometric, cross-correlation technique it is possible to follow spontaneous fluctuations of CBV continuously over time. The rhythmic variations that can be seen in almost all human skin capillaries have been called *flow motion*, and these fluctuations have been studied in both toes and fingers of patients with PAOD (3, 32). As can be seen in **Figure 56**, there is a significant decrease of the flow-motion activity in the diseased digit, probably because of the vasodilatation induced in ischemic regions. The prevalence of flow motion in toes of patients with PAOD has been found to be significantly (p<0.05) lower (25%) than in healthy subjects (80%), but the frequency is similar (4.5–5.5 cycles/min) (3).

With the laser Doppler method for studying the total skin microcirculation, flow-motion waves with a frequency of ≈20 cycles/min have been found in patients with PAOD at a succesively higher (33→92%) prevalence with the

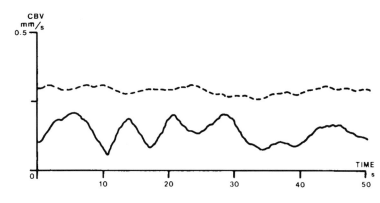

Figure 56. CBV recordings from one single nailfold capillary in a healthy subject. Solid line represent the CBV at a temperature of 25.2°C, and the dashed line is the CBV at a temperature of 33.2°C. The flow motion variations are almost completely abolished at the higher skin temperature because of vasodilatation.

severity of ischemia (37). Such fast flow-motion waves have never been seen in the CBV tracings, which could mean that they do not exist in these vessels, or that the cross-correlation technique is not sensitive enough to record these fast components.

Comments: Vasomotion is an activity of the smoth muscle cells in the vascular walls and seems to be most prominent at the level of the arterioles of tissues. Its activity is centrally mediated through hormones and the nervous system, and locally controlled by myogenic mechanisms. It is present in the the skin microcirculation to optimize the regulation of blood flow in different vascular compartments of the skin microcirculation, and to regulate tissue nutrition and fluid exchange. The activity is markedly changed in pathological conditions, and it may be of importance for the treatment of the microvascular disturbances if vasmotion activity could be restored (20).

Fluorescent Dyes

Distribution of skin perfusion at the *macroscopic level* has been studied with NaF (26, 29, 34). These investigations are based on the observation that the dye reaches low flow areas with delay and does not color areas with stagnant flow. For practical purposes, the technique has been used to detect regions with particularly impaired flow (26, 34) and to predict adequate amputation levels (29).

Mapping skin areas by intravital microscopy as described above is a well-established method for predicting the healing of lesions in ischemic skin (10, 14) that does not require injection of a dye. It is used by preference in smaller areas like the forefoot, whereas the fluorescent technique at the macroscopic level is a better alternative for investigating larger parts of extremities.

To our knowledge, only one major study has used fluorescent dyes at the *microvascular level* (23). The results obtained contribute to the understanding of pathophysiology in chronic ischemia and may form a basis for investigations of therapy control. It should be remembered that chronic human ischemia is by no means comparable to the conditions present in ischemic animal preparations where acute conditions prevail (16, 38).

The pathophysiologic phenomena involving microcirculation in chronic skin ischemia are complex. In the low-pressure area distal to arterial obstructions (2), microvessels often exhibit pathologic flux motion, as demonstrated by laser Doppler fluxmetry (37). The prevalence of flux motion waves with a frequency of about 21 cycles/min increases with the degree of ischemia. Moreover, microvascular dynamics critically depend on limb position (19). In severe foot ischemia, reflex vasoconstriction in the upright or sitting position is reduced or abolished.

Microvascular flow distribution and transcapillary diffusion were studied at the forefoot

Figure 57. Image of capillaries at the foot dorsum appearing as dots in a patient with incipient gangrene. The numbers indicate time elapsed since NaF injection in the arm.
(a) and (b): Late and inhomogeneous filling of capillaries by NaF.
(c) and (d): Prompt and homogeneous filling of the same capillaries one day after successful peripheral transluminal angioplasty.
(e): Densitometer evaluation of microvascular perfusion on a horizontal axis crossing the observation field (severe ischemia before transluminal angioplasty). The peaks correspond to loops reached by the dye. Only 1 min 30 s after first arrival of NaF, all the capillaries are perfused (inhomogeneous perfusion).

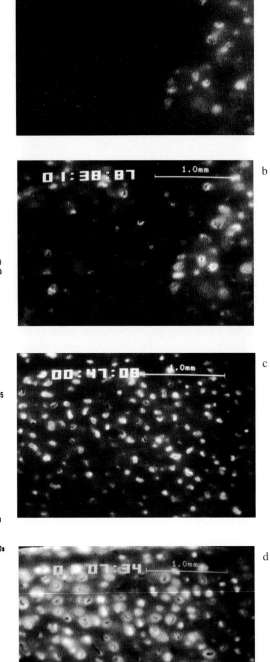

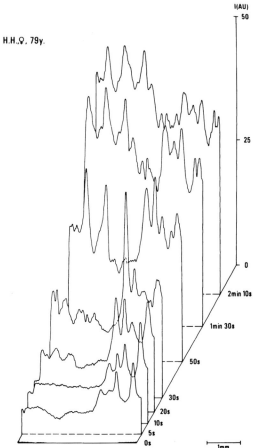

Table 13. Mean appearance time (A) and time interval between first and last capillary filling (I) in normals (n = 21), patients with intermittent claudication (n = 35) and patients with rest pain or incipient gangrene (n = 29) according to Jünger et al. (23).

	A	I
Normals	53.4±15.7 s (23–82 s)	23.2±7.6 s (12–48 s)
Intermittent claudication	53.1±16.4 s (30–101 s)	29.9±12.1 s* (12–63 s)
Rest pain or gangrene	57.5±27.1 s (22–155 s)	31.5±14.2 s* (12–71 s)

* significant difference to normal mean value (p < 0.05)

in 21 healthy volunteers, 35 patients with chronic intermittent claudication, and 29 patients with chronic rest pain or incipient gangrene (23). The corresponding mean systolic arm/ankle pressure ratios were 1.18 ± 0.07, 0.71 ± 0.16, and 0.38 ± 0.19, respectively. The results are described below.

Inhomogeneity of Microvascular Perfusion

The appearance time of NaF at the forefoot just proximal to the first and second toe was not different between controls and patients with moderate and severe ischemia, although range and standard deviation was largest in patients with rest pain and gangrene (**Table 13**). One possible explanation for this surprising fact is that the longer distance the dye travels through the collateral vessels is compensated by the well-known dilatation of the arterioles in ischemic areas. Findings in patients with occlusions of hand and finger arteries not resulting from collagen vascular disease support this view (15).

In contrast to appearance time, the time interval between the first and last filling of the capillaries in the visualized field of 2.8 mm^2 was significantly ($p<0.05$) prolonged in patients (**Table 13**), indicating inhomogeneous microvascular perfusion in chronic limb ischemia. Video microscopic images at different times after first dye appearance in a patient with severe ischemia illustrate the inhomogeneous inflow of dye that was normalized one day after successful peripheral transluminal angioplasty of a short femoral artery occlusion (**Figure 57**).

Transcapillary Diffusion of NaF

In the same controls and patients (23), transcapillary diffusion of NaF was measured in a rectangular skin area of the forefoot (2.8 mm^2). The mean values were significantly enhanced in both patient groups (**Table 14**). Especially high values were observed in diabetic patients with

Table 14. Mean values and standard deviations of fluorescent light intensities (23) during 10 minutes after first dye appearance (percentage of peak intensity in each subject). Values in parenthesis: number of capillaries in the field of observation (2.8 mm^2).

Time	Controls (109±14) 39/mm^2	Moderate ischemia (95±29) 34/mm^2	Severe ischemia (88±23) 31/mm^2	Severe ischemia nondiabetics	Severe ischemia diabetics
5 s	2.8± 3.1	3.0± 4.4	4.5± 4.0	3.3± 2.8	5.7± 4.7
10 s	3.9± 3.6	5.1± 5.1	9.5± 8.7*+	6.2± 6.4	13.1± 9.6
30 s	11.6± 6.5	16.5± 9.9	29.1±21.4*+	18.5±14.5	40.5±22.3°*
60 s	20.4± 7.4	28.5± 9.5*	44.7±21.3*+	31.2±16.7*	59.3±15.5°*
2 min	35.9± 9.3	43.7±10.8	60.3±20.4*+	46.8 ±15.1*	74.7±14.7°*
5 min	66.0±11.9	72.6±16.2	84.7±15.7*+	77.6±16.2	92.3±11.3°*
10 min	91.8± 7.0	92.2± 7.4	91.1±11.4	94.2± 8.1	87.1±14.1

* significant difference in comparison to the controls ($p<0.05$–0.01)
+ significant difference between moderate and severe ischemia ($p<0.05$–0.001)
° significant difference between the diabetics and nondiabetics with severe ischemia ($p<0.05$–0.001)

Chapter 2.1

Figure 58. "Candle-light phenomenon" at the dorsum of the foot in a patient with severe ischemia. Some of the capillaries (dark dots or commas) embedded in slightly fluorescing halos carry bright fluorescent spots at their apex corresponding to preferential sites of dye leakage.

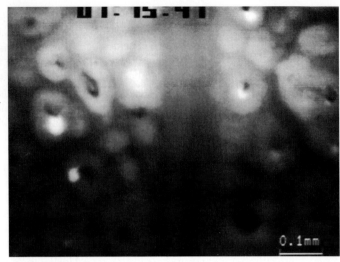

Figure 59. Prevalence of "candle-light phenomenon" in controls (n = 21), patients with moderate (n = 35) and severe (n = 29) ischemia at the foot dorsum (from Jünger et al., 23).

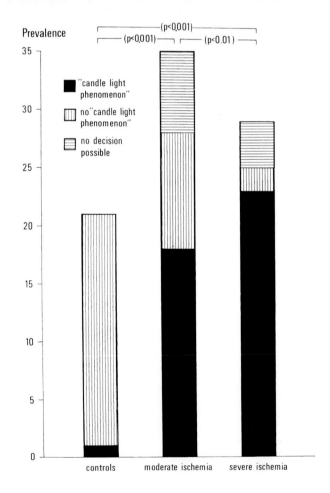

severe ischemia (see page 87). Increased transcapillary diffusion was measured although the number of capillaries containing red cells tended to be lower in the patients than in the controls (**Table 14**). However, there might have been a certain number of capillaries filled by plasma alone. The relatively low magnification required for measurement of transcapillary diffusion in skin areas did not allow distinction between plasma- and erythrocyte-filled microvessels.

After the end of transcapillary diffusion measurements, the capillaries of the forefoot were examined by a large magnification. The loops appearing as dots or commas were embedded in a circular pericapillary halo stained by NaF. Some of the capillaries exhibited spots of high fluorescent light intensity at their apex (**Figure 58**). Because of the visual impression evoked, the finding was called *candle light phenomenon*. Its prevalence was significantly ($p<0.001$) enhanced in patients with moderate and severe ischemia (**Figure 59**). It probably develops in capillary loops particularly damaged by ischemia and corresponds to preferential sites of dye leakage. The phenomenon occurred more frequently in patients with severe than with moderate ischemia. The observation that pigmentation from extravasation of erythrocytes is common in severe ischemia (10, 14) fits well into the concept of localized spots of increased NaF diffusion.

In conclusion, arterial ischemia from chronic peripheral arterial occlusive disease induces enhanced transcapillary diffusion of NaF at the single capillary level (candle light phenomenon) and in forefoot skin areas. Pathologic changes of the capillary wall were detected by electron microscopy (16, 17). They may explain that the capillary wall becomes a less tight barrier for NaF diffusion. With increasing duration of ischemia, the endothelial cells swell and lose their integrity. These alterations affect some capillaries more than others, perhaps explaining the patchy distribution of capillaries with preferential sites of leakage. A further reason for increased transcapillary diffusion may be the loss of autoregulation in severe ischemia (7, 19). According to Levick and Michel (25), the filtration rate augments 13 times when autoregulation is almost abolished.

Moreover, there is increasing evidence that leucocytes block microvessels under conditions of low perfusion pressure and become activated (31). When they are trapped in the microcirculation, they may trigger damage to the microvessel walls and initiate increased permeability (24, 35).

Control of Therapy

Measurements one day after successful reopening of large obstructed arteries by peripheral transluminal angioplasty revealed a prompt and significant ($p<0.01$) increase in fluorescent light intensity in identical skin areas of the forefoot (unpublished data). Transcapillary diffusion was still more enhanced than before treatment (**Figure 60**). This finding correlates to postischemic edema, which often develops after reconstructive vascular surgery or peripheral transluminal angioplasty. Transcutaneous oxygen tension was only marginally improved one day after catheter therapy. Oxygen diffusion seems to be impaired during postischemic edema. It normalized only during the following weeks. Similarly, transcapillary diffusion dropped to almost normal values within a month after the reopening procedure (**Figure 60**).

At least in part, the increase of transcapillary diffusion after successful therapy results from augmented skin flow. Postischemic hyperemia is a well-known phenomenon after recanalization of proximal arteries (39, 40). Arteriolar dilatation is responsible for elevated capillary blood pressure contributing to fluid extravasation (5). Even macromolecular permeability is enhanced in the postischemic state (8, 33). FITC-labeled dextran 150,000 leaks out of postcapillary venules at an increased number of sites, as demonstrated in the hamster's cheek pouch preparation. The β_2-receptor antagonist terbutaline abolishes the permeability response to ischemia (8). Again, the leucocytes appear to be crucial for the development of reperfusion damage (24, 35). When ischemic tissue is reperfused by blood depleted of leucocytes, the

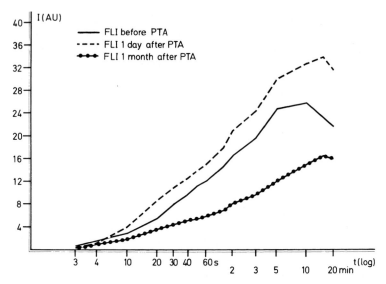

Figure 60. a) Mean intensity of fluorescence light (arbitrary units: AU) 20 s after first dye appearance and monitored at the dorsum of the foot in 30 patients with intermittent claudication (n = 18) or rest pain with or without gangrene (n = 12) before, 1 day after, and 1 month after peripheral transluminal angioplasty (PTA) of iliac or femoro-popliteal arteries. Time is plotted on a logarithmic scale. The mean values before treatment are significantly enhanced compared to healthy controls, but still increase 1 day after successful reopening of proximal arteries (p<0.01). The lowest values are recorded at the control 1 month later (Jünger).

b) Densitometer curves recorded by the large window technique after NaF injection at the forefoot of a patient with severe ischemia before and after successful transluminal angioplasty. After reopening of the vessels, fluorescent light intensity increases much steeper than before catheter treatment.

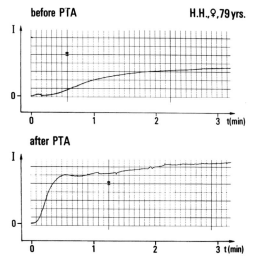

vascular injury is attenuated. In addition, oxygen-derived free radicals appear to play an important role in postischemic microvascular injury (1, 27). The different factors interact in a way not yet fully understood.

References 2.1

1) Ambrosio, G., Weisfeldt, M. L., Jacobus, W. E. Flaherty, J. R.: Evidence for a reversible oxygen radical-mediated component of reperfusion injury: reduction by recombinant human superoxide dismutase administered at the time of reflow. *Circulation* 75, 282–291, 1987.

2) Bollinger, A., Barras, J. P., Mahler, F.: Measurement of foot artery blood pressure by micromanometry in normal subjects and in patients with arterial occlusive disease. *Circulation* 53, 506–512, 1976.

3) Bongard, O., Fagrell, B.: Discrepancies between total and nutritional skin microcirculation in patients with peripheral arterial

occlusive disease (PAOD). *VASA* 19, 105–111, 1990.

4) Conrad, M. C.: Abnormalities of the digital vasculature as related to ulceration and gangrene. *Circulation* 88, 568–581, 1968.

5) Diana, J. N., Laughlin, M. H.: Effect of ischemia on capillary pressure and equivalent pore radius in capillaries of the isolated dog hind limb. *Circ. Res.* 35, 77–101, 1974.

6) Davis, E., Landau, J.: *Clinical capillary microscopy.* Charles C. Thomas, Springfield, IL, U.S.A., 1966

7) Eickhoff, J. H.: Normalization of local blood flow regulation in the ischemic forefoot after arterial reconstruction. *Surgery* 97, 72–81, 1985.

8) Erlansson, M., Persson, N. H., Svensjö, E., Bergqvist, D.: Macromolecular permeability increases following incomplete ischemia in the hamster cheek pouch and its inhibition by terbutaline. *Int. J. Microcir.: Clin. Exp.* 6, 265–271, 1987.

9) Fagrell, B.: Vital capillaroscopy–A clinical method for studying changes of skin microcirculation in patients suffering from vascular disorders of the leg. *Angiology* 23, 284–298, 1972.

10) Fagrell, B.: Vital capillary microscopy—A clinical method for studying changes of the nutritional skin capillaries in legs with arteriosclerosis obliterans. *Scand. J. Clin. Lab. Invest.*, Suppl. 133, 1973.

11) Fagrell, B.: The skin microcirculation and the pathogenis of ischemic necrosis and gangrene. *Scand. J. Clin. Lab. Invest.* 37, 473–476, 1977.

12) Fagrell, B.: Structual changes of human skin capillaries in chronic arterial and venous insufficiency. *Bibl. Anat.* 20, 645–648, 1981.

13) Fagrell, B., Lund, F.: Vital capillary microscopy as a test method for therapeutic procedures in peripheral vascular diseases. In: *Clinical evaluation of testing methods of vasoactive drugs effects*, pp. 329–334, C.E.P.I. Rome, 1968.

14) Fagrell, B., Lundberg, G.: A simplified evaluation of vital capillary microscopy for predicting skin viability in patients with severe arterial insufficiency. *Clin. Physiol.* 4, 403–411, 1984.

15) Franzeck, U. K., Isenring, G., Frey, J., Bollinger, A.: Video densitometric pattern recognition of Na-fluorescein diffusion in nailfold capillary areas of patients with acrocyanosis, primary vasospastic and secondary Raynaud's phenomenon. *Inter. Angio.* 2, 143–152, 1983.

16) Gidlöff, A., Larsson, J., Lewis, D., Hammersen, F.: Capillary endothelial alterations affecting reperfusion after ischemia in human skeletal muscle. *Biblthca. Anat.* 20, 572–577, 1981.

17) Gidlöff, A., Lewis, D. H., Hammersen, F.: The effect of prolonged total ischemia on the ultrastructure of human skeletal muscle capillaries. A morphometric analysis. *Int. J. Microcirc.: Clin. Exp.* 7, 67–86, 1987.

18) Heisig, N.: Untersuchungen über das mikrovaskuläre System bei degenerativen Gefässkrankungen. *Arch. Kreisl.-Forsch* 47, 95–137, 1965.

19) Henriksen, O.: Orthostatic changes of blood flow in subcutaneous tissue in patients with arterial insufficiency of the legs. *Scand. J. Clin. Lab. Invest.* 34, 103–109, 1974.

20) Intaglietta, M.: Arteriolar vasomotion: Normal physiological activity or defense mechanism? *Diabète & Metabolisme* 14, 489–494, 1988.

21) Jogestrand, T., Berglund, B.: Estimation of digital circulation and its correlation to clinical signs of ischaemia—A comparative methodological study. *Clin. Physiol.* 3, 307–312, 1983.

22) Johnson, P. C., Burton, K. S., Henrich, H.: Effect of occlusion duration on reactive hyperemia in sartorius muscle capillaries. *Am. J. Physiol.* 230(3), 715–719, 1976.

23) Jünger, M., Frey-Schnewlin, G., Bollinger, A.: Microvascular flow distribution and transcapillary diffusion at the forefoot in patients with peripheral ischemia. *Int. J. Microcirc.: Clin. Exp.* 8, 3–24, 1989.

24) Korthuis, R. J., Grisham, M. B., Granger, D. N.: Leukocyte depletion attenuates vascular injury in postischemic skeletal muscle. *Am. J. Physiol.* 254, H823–H827, 1988.

25) Levick, J. R., Michel, C. C.: The effects of position and skin temperature on the capil-

lary pressure in fingers and toes. *J. Physiol.* (London) 274, 97–108, 1978.
26) Lund, F.: Dynamic fluorescence angiography for evaluating occlusive arterial disease of the limbs and for assessing increased microvascular permeability of the skin. In L. A. Carlson (ed.): *Int. Conf. on Atherosclerosis.* Raven Press, New York, 429–439, 1978.
27) McCord, J. M.: Oxygen-derived free radicals in postischemic tissue injury. *New Engl. J. Med.* 312, 159–163, 1985.
28) McEvan, A., Ledingham, I.: Blood flow characteristics and tissue nutrition in apparently ischaemic feet. *Br. Med. J.* 3, 220–224, 1971.
29) McFarland, D. C., Lawrence, P. F.: Skin fluorescence, a method to predict amputation site healing. *J. Surg. Res.* 32, 410–415, 1982.
30) Morris-Jones, W., Preston, E., Greaney, M., Duleep, K.: Gangrene of the toes with palpable peripheral pulses. *Ann. Surg.* 193, 462–466, 1981.
31) Nash, G. B., Thomas, P. R. S., Dormandy, J. A.: Abnomal flow properties of white blood cells in patients with severe ischemia of the leg. *Brit. Med. J.* 296, 1699–1701, 1988.
32) Östergren, J., Fagrell, B.: Skin capillary blood cell velocity in patients with arterial obliterative disease and polycythemia—A disturbed reactive hyperemia response. *Clin. Physiol.* 5, 35–43, 1985.
33) Persson, N. H., Erlansson, M., Svensjö, E., Takolander, R., Bergqvist, D.: The hamster cheek pouch—an experimental model to study macromolecular permeability. *Int. J. Microcir.: Clin. Exp.* 4, 257–263, 1985.
34) Scheffler, A., Rieger, H.: Einfluß einer hydrostatischen Druckerhöhung auf die Fluoreszenz-Erscheinungszeitverteilungsmuster bei Patienten mit peripherer arterieller Verschlußkrankheit. VASA, Suppl. 27, 228–230, 1989.
35) Schmid-Schönbein, G. W.: Capillary plugging by granulocytes and the no reflow phenomenon in the microcirculation. *Fed. Proc.* 46, 2397–2401, 1987.
36) Schwartz, R. W., Freedman, A. M., Richardson, D. R., Hyde, G. L., Griffen, W. O., Vincent, D. G., Price, M. A.: Capillary blood flow: Video densitometry in the atherosclerotic patient. *J. Vasc. Surg.* 1, 800–808, 1984.
37) Seifert, H., Jäger, K., Bollinger, A.: Analysis of flow motion by the laser Doppler technique in patients with peripheral arterial occlusive disease. *Int. J. Microcirc.: Clin. Exp.* 7, 223–236, 1988.
38) Slaaf, D. W., Tangelder, G. J., Teirlinck, H. C., Reneman, R. S.: Arteriolar vasomotion and arterial pressure reduction in rabbit tenuissimus muscle. *Microvasc. Res.* 33, 71–80, 1987.
39) Stranden, E., Myhre, H. O.: Pressure-volume recordings of human subcutaneous tissue: A study in patients with edema following arterial reconstruction for lower limb atherosclerosis. *Microvasc. Res.* 24, 241–248, 1982.
40) Stranden, E.: Transcapillary fluid filtration in patients with leg edema following arterial reconstruction for lower limb atherosclerosis. *VASA* 12, 219–224, 1983.

2.2 Diabetes

Diabetes mellitus, whether insulin dependent or not, is associated with increased prevalence of macro- and microangiopathy. Whereas stenoses and occlusions developing in large arteries cannot be clearly separated from atherosclerotic lesions of other origin, microangiopathy is quite characteristic for the disease. It primarily involves retinal and renal vessels. At the foot, where macroangiopathy, neuropathy, and infection may contribute to the clinical picture, the role of microangiopathy is less established (31). In this chapter, evidence is presented that diabetic microvascular disease is important also in the skin and might be one of the determining factors in the diabetic foot.

Table 15 reviews the most important events during the development of diabetic microangiopathy. Some steps remain hypothetical at present. First, hyperglycemia induces metabolic changes in endothelial cells, basement membranes, and vascular smooth muscles. When they concern the contractile properties of the arteriolar wall, microvascular hemodynamics are altered. Changes at the capillary and possibly venular level elicit increased permeability. At this early stage the alterations are reversible.

Later on, the microvessels lose their elasticity and are transformed into stiff conduits with increased wall thickness (5). Microaneurysms and microvascular occlusions may develop. Then major and only partially reversible or irreversible disturbances of microvascular hemodynamics and permeability occur. Organ failure is the ultimate result.

Anatomical and Biochemical Changes

Hyperglycemia induces biochemical changes. Two main pathways that are most probably linked with each other have been described as inducing damage of microvascular walls: non-

Table 15. Hypothetical cascade of main events during development of diabetic microangiopathy.

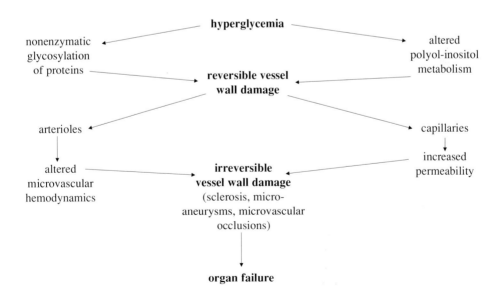

enzymatic glycosylation of proteins (5) and *altered polyol-inositol metabolism* (19, 54).

Glucose forms chemically reversible early glycosylation products with protein which in part undergo a complex rearrangement to form irreversible advanced glycosylation end products. In contrast to the reversible ones, these latter products accumulate during the lifetime of vessels wall proteins. The rate of this accumulation is proportional to the time-integrated blood glucose level over long periods of time. In diabetics larger amounts of advanced glycosylation end products are observed in various tissues including arterial walls and basement membranes (5).

A specific macrophage receptor recognizes proteins to which advanced glycosylation end products are bound and stimulates their removal (5). The interaction initiates a cascade of events with formation of interleukin-1 and tumor necrosis factor. The latter substance appears to induce dysfunction of the endothelial cells and extracellular matrix, thus favoring enhanced permeability. The negatively charged proteoglycans contained in the basement membranes are decreased in diabetics, thus probably rendering them more permeable.

Since the amount of vascular wall proteins is increased by end-product accumulation (reduced enzymatic degradation), the wall thickens and becomes inelastic. This pathway of damage is probably responsible for the changes of microvascular hemodynamics described below.

The second biochemical alteration that is well documented to damage the nerve fibers and walls of microvessels concerns the so-called *polyol-inositol pathway* (19, 54). In hyperglycemia, free intracellular glucose is increased, stimulating activity of the polyol pathway and depleting pools of myo-inositol. As a consequence, Na^+-K^+-ATPase regulation is deranged. This particular ATPase is involved in plasma membrane transport and therefore in microvascular function. Hence, it is assumed that glomerular hemodynamics are affected by these changes. Decreased Na^+-K^+-ATPase activity influences the contraction of vascular smooth muscle. Moreover, increased accumulation of Na-fluorescein in the vitreous of diabetics has been explained by altered polyol metabolism (54).

Both biochemical cascades of events induced by hyperglycemia are bases for new pharmacologic attempts to block development of microangiopathy at an early reversible stage. Aldose reductase inhibitors could block increased polyol pathway activity (19, 54) and aminoguanidine the formation of advanced glycosylation end products (5).

The salient anatomical finding in diabetic microangiopathy is a *thickening of the capillary basement membrane* (51), which is composed of a latticework of type IV collagen, laminin, and a negatively charged heparin sulphate proteoglycan as well as of other unique proteins. It has been demonstrated in most of the organs and tissues of the body. Thickening of basement membrane is particularly enhanced in the lower leg, where diameters are even increased in normal subjects compared to other regions of the body (39).

Morphological studies of *endothelial cells* have failed to show any characteristic anomalies. On the other hand, acellular capillaries have been detected frequently in diabetics (39).

A phenomenon studied in the retina is capillary *neogenesis*: Sprouts of newly formed capillaries grow into nonperfused areas (36). The capacity of the endothelial cells to synthesize important biochemical substances is altered in diabetes. Von Willebrand factor, for example, circulates in increased amounts in the plasma of patients (36).

Pericytes, which are supposed to be involved in regulating the size of interendothelial cell junctions and to influence permeability, degenerate more rapidly in diabetic patients than in normals (39, 46). The regeneration capacity of these still enigmatic cells keeps pace with accelerated degeneration (39).

Intravital Capillary Morphology

Intravital microscopy of nailfold capillaries does not reveal striking changes. There is no

Diabetes

loss or evident enlargement of loops like in microangiopathy because of progressive systemic sclerosis (see page 122).

Significant changes are found only in large patient samples examined by morphometric methods or by classifying loop morphology. Prevalence of coiled and slightly enlarged microvessels is significantly increased in long-term diabetics at the nailfold of fingers (32, 37) and toes (6, 32). Slim capillary loops are present both in normals and diabetics, but the prevalence is lower in the patients. An inverse distribution is found for widened loops, which occur more frequently in diabetics.

The width of the capillary loops has been determined at the end-row of the nailfold. It corresponds to the maximal distance between the outer contours of the arterial and venous limb of a given loop. In long-term diabetics with a mean disease duration of 19 years, mean loop diameter was 46.0 ± 22.4 µm, in controls only 42.5 ± 14.7 µm (32). Because of the large number of loops studied (>3000), this relatively small difference was statistically significant ($p<0.001$).

It is interesting to note that the mean diameter of toe nailfold loops is significantly larger than the mean width of the finger loops, suggesting a modeling effect of hydrostatic factors. In 50-year-old controls and patients, mean loop width at the foot was 64.3 ± 43.5 µm and 76.0 ± 46.1 µm, respectively. At the foot dorsum, areas containing dilated capillaries were more common in long-term diabetics on oral drugs ($p<0.05$) and on insulin ($p<0.01$) than in age-matched controls (13).

The morphological changes described are not sufficiently pronounced to be used diagnostically for diabetic microangiopathy in single cases. However, they may be useful for characterizing patient samples. Correlations between morphologic and functional alterations will be important in the future.

Similar changes of capillary morphology have been described in the conjunctiva (7, 12, 55). In particular, the venules were enlarged and the density of microvessels decreased. A precise morphometric study (17) confirmed reduced conjunctival microvessel density, but this parameter was as well correlated to age as to the presence or absence of diabetes.

Changes in Microvascular Dynamics

Microcirculation is known to be disturbed in many organs of diabetic patients. It has been shown with different methods that the dynamics of microvascular flow regulation in the skin is impaired, but only a few studies have been performed where the blood flow of the skin capillaries were investigated in humans. Some of these results are presented here.

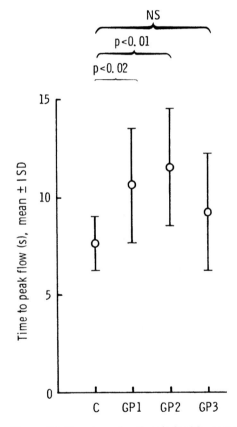

Figure 61. Time to peak values in healthy controls subjects (C), type 1 diabetics with a duration of <1 year (GP 1), and with a duration of >10 years (GP 2). Group 3 (GP 3) represents patients similar to those in GP 2, but with an HbA1 persistantly less than 9% (= good control).

Changes in Type 1 Diabetics

During the past decade, significant changes in skin capillary blood flow have been described in diabetics (42, 45). In one study, CBV was recorded in three groups of Type 1 diabetic patients (42). Group 1 had a diabetes duration of less than 1 year; Group 2 approximately 10 years duration; and Group 3 was similar to Group 2 but had a HbA_{1c} persistantly less than 9% (= well controlled). One healthy control group of nondiabetics was also investigated (C in **Figure 61**).

It was found that resting CBV did not differ significantly in patients with diabetes as compared to controls, which is in agreement with the findings in another study (13). However, the time to pCBV after 60 s of arterial occlusion was significantly (p<0.01) increased in the patients with both short and long durations (**Figure 61**). In patients with optimal control of the diabetes (Group 3), the time to pCBV was improved and did not differ significantly from the control subjects. This finding indicates that the reactivity of the skin precapillary vessels can be improved if the diabetic control is optimized, also in patients with long-standing diabetes.

In another study (20), in which patients with diabetes of more than 10 years' duration and severe macro- and microvascular complications were investigated, resting CBV was only 0.15 ± 0.10 mm/s, which was significantly (p<0.01) lower than in age- and sex-matched controls (0.46 ± 0.35 mm/s). The reason for this low CBV may have been a significantly lower skin temperature in the patients than in the controls, though it was found that it was mainly the patients with the highest skin temperature who had a significantly lower resting CBV than the healthy controls. The low resting CBV at these high skin temperatures may be explained by a redistribution of blood from the nutritional skin capillaries to the subpapillary vascular bed. Such an increased shunt flow has also been shown in previous studies to exist in diabetic patients (4).

When limbs are put into different positions above and below heart level and local blood pressure is adjusted accordingly, autoregulation is impaired in diabetic patients with microangiopathy (24). Depressed vasodilator responses of precapillary resistance vessels in human skin have also been documented by local clearance of radioisotopes (25).

The decrease of microvascular response to circulatory arrest or venous occlusion was not very marked in a group with excellent HbA_{1c} levels (48). Consequently, optimal adjustment of glycemia seems to prevent or reverse in part decreased microvascular reactivity.

The Effect of Insulin on CBV in Type 1 Diabetics

There is considerable evidence that the development of diabetic microangiopathy relates to the degree and duration of hyperglycemia, but little is know about the influence of insulin on skin capillary function. Tooke et al. (41) investigated the effects of insulin infusion (1.5 µU/h and 15 µU/h) on finger CBV both during rest, after 60 s of arterial occlusion, and during 30 s of venous occlusion. Blood glucose was maintained constant at preinfusion values by intravenous glucose infusion.

There was a successive increase in the capillary (i.e., the erythrocyte column) diameter in the nailfold capillaries, both at the arterial and venous end, although the diameter only increased significantly at the highest insulin infusion rate and in the venous limb. The resting CBV did not change at all on insulin infusion, though as the erythrocyte column diameter was increased, the total capillary blood flow increased. The postocclusive reactive hyperemia showed a significant increase when insulin was infused. During venous occlusion, CBV fell significantly more on the physiological concentration of insulin and went back to prelevel on the hyperphysiological dose.

Comments: The results demonstrate that insulin sometimes may have a clear effect on skin capillary dynamics in Type 1 diabetics. Since the glucose levels were kept almost constant during the study procedure, hyperglycemia could not have attributed to the changes seen. The resting CBV was not significantly changed, but the relative capillary volume flow was increased on the high dose insulin infusion. As it has been shown that the total skin microcirculation, as evaluated, for example, by laser Doppler fluxmetry, is reduced during high dose insulin infusion (41), it seems as if insulin may induce a redistribution of peripheral microcirculatory flow in favor of the nutritive capillary circulation, which may have clinical implications.

Effect of Combined Pancreas and Kidney Transplantation (CPKT) on CBV

The best way to adjust the hyperglycemia to normoglycemia in diabetics is by pancreas transplantation. Normoglycemia is then mostly instituted within 24 hours and the patients do not need to take insulin. The CBV has been measured in diabetics with severe late complications before and 12 months after CPKT. The results were compared with those obtained in a similar group of diabetic patients waiting for CPKT, and healthy age- and sex-matched control subjects (20). It was found that CBV at rest and during postocclusive hyperemia was significantly reduced in both patient groups as compared to the healthy controls. However, the time to peak CBV during hyperemia was normal in the posttransplantation group, but significantly prolonged before transplantation as compared to healthy controls (**Figure 62**). The ability to decrease flow during venous stasis, the so-called veno-arteriolar reflex, was also strongly impaired in the pretransplantation group but less so after transplantation.

Comments: The results show that there is a tendency toward better microvascular reactivity in the nutritional skin capillaries of diabetic patients who have undergone CPKT, and it is encouraging that some variables do not differ from those in healthy controls, which may indicate that the normalized blood glucose level after CPKT can institute a regression of microvascular disturbances. However, most of the patients investigated had serious macro- and microvascular complications and had most probably already passed the state at which the microangiopathy can be reversed by normalization of the glucose metabolism. The observation period may also have been to short (12 months) for recovery of the damage, since it has been shown that it may take up to 2 years of near normoglucemia before any effects on diabetic retinopathy or incipient neuropathy can be observed (11, 29). The investigated patients are now being reinvestigated 4 years after the CPKT in order to study whether further improvement of the skin precapillary reactivity has taken place.

Effect of Kidney Transplantation on CBV

In order to rule out that the positive effect recorded in the CBV reactivity after CPKT did

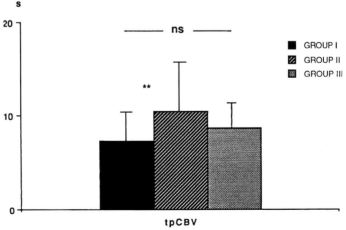

Figure 62. Time to peak CBV (tpCBV) in healthy controls (Group I), diabetics with severe macro- and microangiopathy waiting for combined pancreas and kidney transplantation (CPKT) (Group II), and patients who had undergone CPKT 20 months prior to the investigation (Group III). The last group showed an improvement of the tpCBV compared to group II (mean ± SD).
**p<0.01

not result from the kidney transplantation, a group of diabetics were also investigated before and after kidney transplantation only. No improvement was recorded after kidney transplantation, which indicates that it is the normoglycemic state after the pancreas, and not the kidney, transplantation that improves skin microcirculation in the CPKT-operated patients (21).

Skin Capillary Pressure in Diabetics

The capillary pressure can be measured in the nailfold capillary loops by *in vivo* microsopy through direct puncture of the capillaries using a microscope and micromanipulators (44). As capillary pressure is not directly a microscopic measurement, we note only that marked changes in skin capillary pressure have been found in diabetic patients (40).

Conclusions

The following *main alterations of microvascular hemodynamics* are found in skin of diabetics:

— Capillary blood cell velocity varies within normal limits during periods of stable metabolic conditions, but may significantly change during periods of intensive treatment or unstable control of glycemia.
— Reaction of precapillary vessel tone to various stimuli is delayed and decreased even in patients with satisfactory long-term treatment. With optimal metabolic control, the changes may be reversible in part.
— There is evidence for redistribution from nutritive to shunt flow during unsatisfactory metabolic situations.
— Insulin influences microvascular reactivity in diabetics.
— Pancreas transplantation may improve the disturbed microvascular reactivity even in a severely damaged cardiovascular system.

Most of these findings are in agreement with the biochemic alterations outlined above and with their functional and morphologic consequences. It makes sense that stiffened arteriolar walls do not react promptly to vasodilator or vasoconstrictor stimuli, and that maximal vasodilatation is decreased and delayed. During the course of the disease the changes become more pronounced, but they are already present during the first year after manifestation. Optimal metabolic control is capable of restoring microvascular reactivity at least in part. This observation fits well into the concept that good therapy improves long-term prognosis.

It is beyond the scope of a book dedicated to capillaroscopy to outline the changes of blood rheology contributing to altered microvascular hemodynamics, particularly under low flow conditions (33, 49).

Permeability

Enhanced capillary permeability to small and large molecules is a well-recognized phenomenon in experimental (8, 22) and clinical (2, 3, 16, 30, 34, 47) diabetes. Most of the results were obtained by using radioisotopes or by dosing microalbuminuria (35). Cunha-Vaz and coworkers introduced a technique to quantitate abnormal penetration of NaF into the vitreous (10), which may be an early sign of retinopathy preceding more severe alterations like microaneurysms or loss of microvessels (50). Direct intravital evidence of increased transcapillary and interstitial diffusion of NaF has been gained in skin microcirculation (3, 18, 38). Fluorescence video microscopy (see page 31) has been applied for studying dynamics of capillary exchange at the single capillary level (3) and in skin areas of the foot dorsum (18, 38).

It is not known whether hemodynamic changes precede changes of permeability, or whether both phenomena develop during the same time period. There are close interrelations between the two pathophysiologic phenomena. For example, increased microvascular flow augments diffusive transport of small solutes through the capillary wall. This latter fact might play a role during the period of hyperperfusion observed early after disease manifestation (43).

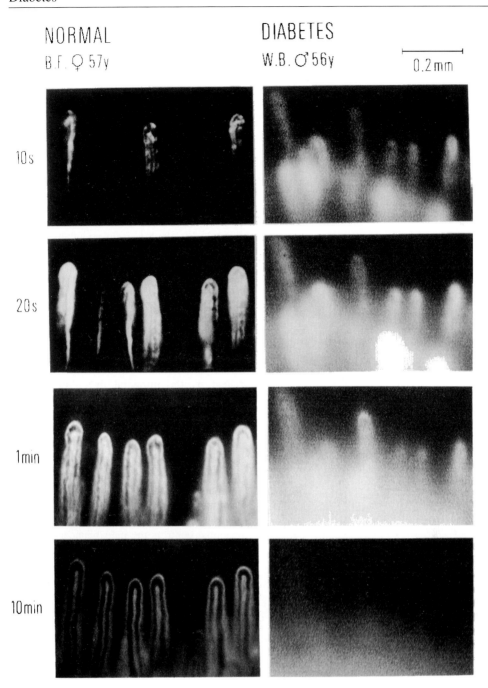

Figure 63. Transcapillary and interstitial diffusion for NaF in nailfold capillaries of a healthy volunteer and a patient with long-term diabetes. In the control, the pericapillary halo is still visible 10 min after dye application, whereas the capillaroscopic image is blurred early in the patient. Photographs were taken on the monitor from single frames of the videotape with constant exposure (by permission from 3).

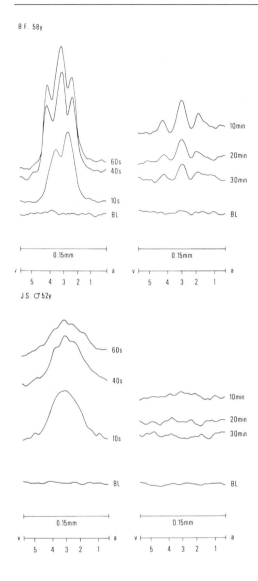

Figure 64. Densitometer curves drawn at various times after NaF appearance in the nailfold capillaries shown in Figure 63.
a) *Healthy control:* The baseline (BL) corresponds to spontaneous fluorescence of the skin. At the halo border steep gradients of fluorescent light intensity are maintained for many minutes. The three peaks correspond to the halo compartment on each side of the loop and the area between the two limbs. Sites 1–5 are identical with those defined in Figure 37.
b) *Long-term diabetic patient:* The steep gradients of light intensities flatten early and move away from the halo border. At 10 min, fluorescence light intensity is evenly distributed around the capillary loop in contrast to the control subject in whom the three peaks remain visible (reprinted by permission from 3).

As has already been described, transcapillary diffusion of NaF through the capillary wall is prompt even in normals (see page 47). A pericapillary halo with well-delineated border is stained by the intravital dye. After having passed the capillary wall, the small dye molecules are confronted with a second diffusion barrier at the outer border of the halo. Both diffusion-limiting structures are significantly more permeable in diabetics than in controls. The dye diffuses in increased amounts through the capillary wall and the outer limit of the halo. The impression of early milky blurring of the microscopic image is created in diabetics, while in normal controls the halo boundary remains well visible for up to 10–20 minutes (**Figure 63**).

The visual findings are objectively assessed by video densitometry. In normals, a steep concentration gradient persists at the halo border for a number of minutes (**Figure 64a**). This gradient of fluorescent light intensity flattens early and moves away from the halo border in long-term diabetic patients (**Figure 64b**). In many instances, the differences of fluorescent light intensity around the capillary loop disappear completely after 5–20 minutes. In healthy controls the normal configuration of the densitometer curve with three peaks is maintained at these late times after dye appearance.

Transcapillary and Interstitial Diffusion of NaF in Single Nailfold Capillaries

Diffusion through the wall of finger nailfold capillaries was studied in 13 long-term diabetics with a mean age of 56 years (mean disease duration of 17 years, 9 patients on insulin, 1 on oral hypoglycemics, and 3 on diet alone) and compared to 12 healthy controls (3). Red blood cell velocity of controls and patients did not differ significantly and was within normal limits.

Table 16. Mean fluorescent light intensities at the nailfold (percentage of peak intensity in each subject) at two sites of measurement defined with respect to the capillary loop and at different times from appearance of NaF (Bollinger et al., 3).

Time	Site 1 Controls	Site 1 Diabetics	Site 2 Controls	Site 2 Diabetics
3 s	8.3± 3.8°	23.3±10.3*°	15.2± 5.5	32.8±18.3*
5 s	12.1± 5.0°	28.1±12.5*°	22.5±10.3	42.0±18.7*
10 s	22.6±11.9°	34.7±13.7*°	43.3±20.7	52.0±19.4
30 s	39.0±12.1°	54.7±10.4*°	61.4±12.2	70.8±17.4
1 min	46.2±10.7°	64.6±11.0*°	65.4±10.1	77.7±12.3*
2 min	54.0± 8.4°	74.4±12.0*°	66.8±13.9	81.5±11.7*
5 min	50.4±12.9°	64.5±11.3*°	58.4±17.8	72.2±15.3
10 min	43.1±18.3°	55.1±12.3*°	48.3±20.7	58.9±14.2
30 min	21.8±11.0°	32.0±10.2*	24.7±12.4	30.8± 8.2
60 min	11.8± 7.4	19.3± 7.6*	12.3± 7.0	18.7± 6.1*

Measurement site 1 was located outside of the halo border, site 2 inside of it next to the capillary wall on the arterial side of the nailfold capillary loop. Data are presented as means and standard deviations.
* differences between controls and diabetics at identical sites were significant ($p<0.01$)
° differences between site 1 and site 2 in controls and diabetics were significant ($p<0.001$)

Table 16 gives the mean values and standard deviations of fluorescent light intensity measured at different times after first arrival of NaF in the nailfold. Significantly increased intensities ($p<0.01$) were determined inside and outside of the halo border, indicating that transcapillary diffusion through the capillary wall and through the outer halo border is increased in long-term diabetics (3). Both diffusion barriers are less effective than in controls. The reduced barrier function of the outer halo limit is also documented by early disappearance of intraindividual concentration gradients at this location. Significant differences between the intra- and extrahalo compartment were measured during the first 10 minutes in diabetics and during 30 minutes in control subjects.

Dye leakage is symmetrical with respect to the arterial and venous limb of the loop. This finding contrasts to asymmetrically enhanced transcapillary and interstitial diffusion in patients with progressive systemic sclerosis (see page 125). Cloud- or street-like accumulations of NaF outside the pericapillary halo are common in scleroderma and uncommon in diabetes.

Transcapillary and Interstitial Diffusion in Skin Areas of the Foot

A second study including exclusively type I diabetics with different disease duration and excluding patients with clinically manifest nephropathy and neuropathy was performed at the dorsum of the foot (38). All patients were in a stable metabolic condition. Fluorescent light intensity was determined in a skin area of 3.2 mm^2 using a relatively small magnification. The field contained a mean number of 120 capillary loops (37/mm^2) appearing as dots or commas. Almost identical capillary density was found in the control group (115 capillaries, 35.5/mm^2).

Like at the nailfold, early blurring of video microscopy images was observed in most patients with diabetes lasting for more than 10 years (**Figure 65**). Single and mean values of fluorescent light intensity are plotted in **Figure 66** for 13 controls, 18 patients with disease duration of less than 10 years, 17 with 10–19 years, and 17 more than 20 years. Significant differences to controls were measured in the last

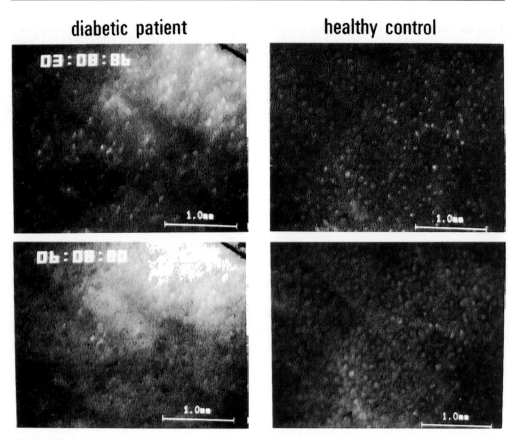

Figure 65.
a) Video microscopic images at the dorsum of the foot in a normal subject and in a patient with long-term type 1 diabetes. At the low magnification used, the small fluorescent dots correspond to the capillary apex and their halo. Early blurring of the image is evident in the patient.

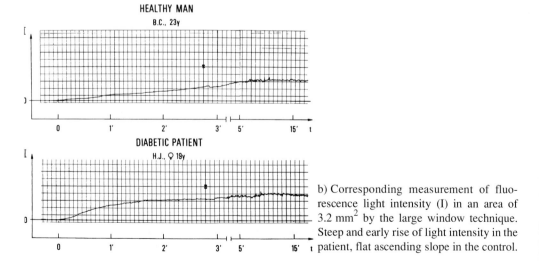

b) Corresponding measurement of fluorescence light intensity (I) in an area of 3.2 mm^2 by the large window technique. Steep and early rise of light intensity in the patient, flat ascending slope in the control.

Diabetes

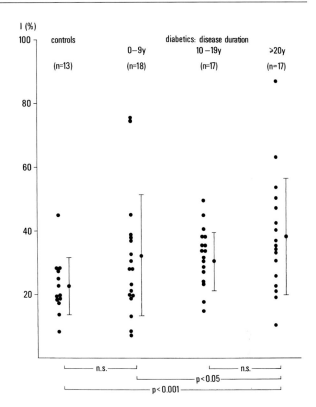

Figure 66. Fluorescence light intensity (I%) 60 s after first dye appearance in a forefoot area (3.0 mm^2) of patients with various duration of type 1 diabetes. Significantly increased transcapillary diffusion was found in patients with disease duration of more than 10 years.

two groups, but not in the group with relatively short duration. It should be noted, however, that fluorescent light intensity in 7 diabetics with short-term disease exceeded the 95% confidence limit of the controls. These patients exhibited increased NaF diffusion before reaching 10 years of disease duration. On the other hand, the values determined in long-term disease are not elevated in each patient. It is not known whether enhanced transcapillary diffusion in a given patient carries an increased risk for developing microvascular complications.

Correlations between fluorescent light intensity at a given time after dye arrival, HbA$_{1c}$, and glucose levels were not significant. Therefore, short-term control of metabolism does not significantly influence the readings. It must be realized that the groups of patients studied were well treated by insulin, since mean HbA$_{1c}$ levels were 6.6%, 7.2%, and 7.3% in the three cohorts with short, middle, and long disease duration. No studies including patients with unsatisfactory metabolic control, with severe neuropathy, and/or nephropathy have been performed yet.

It has been described in a previous chapter (see page 71) that transcapillary diffusion of NaF at the forefoot is enhanced in ischemia because of peripheral arterial occlusive disease. A significant difference ($p<0.001$) was found between diabetics and nondiabetics in patients with incipient gangrene (23). Although scattering of individual values of light intensity was considerable because of the heterogeneity of clinical features in severe ischemia, mean transcapillary diffusion was considerably higher in the diabetic than in the nondiabetic patients (see **Table 14**, page 71). The increased prevalence of infection in the diabetics most probably contributes to enhanced dye leakage.

Comments

Studies with fluorescence video microscopy have the advantage over investigations using radioactive tracers that they provide direct comparison between microvascular anatomy and visualized diffusion of fluorescent dyes. Fluorescent light intensities may be determined by densitometry in well-defined tissue compartments. It is important to realize that flow determines, in part, the transcapillary and interstitial diffusion of small solutes. In the first study (3), capillary red blood cell velocities were almost identical, and in the second (38) metabolic control was excellent, so that there was no reason for increased microvascular blood flow at the dorsum of the foot. The number of capillaries contributing to pericapillary fluorescent light intensity is also easily counted. It did not differ significantly between controls and diabetics.

It cannot be excluded that some coupling of NaF occurs in the interstitial space and influences propagation of the dye. The amount of free NaF in plasma is slightly lower in diabetics than in controls (27). Therefore, differences of plasma protein binding of NaF cannot account for increased transcapillary diffusion of the dye. The best explanation for increased diffusion into the halo and the more remote interstitial space is partial breakdown of the diffusion barrier function exerted by the capillary wall and the halo border (3, 38).

If it is accepted that pericytes contribute to regulate fluid exchange across the capillary wall, the degeneration of these cells (39) could account in part for increased permeability. Moreover, the accumulation of irreversible glucosylation end products could be responsible for the altered diffusion capacity of the membranes involved (5).

Compared to the penetration of NaF into the vitreous as an early sign of diabetic retinopathy (10), increased transcapillary and interstitial diffusion of the same fluorescent compound appears to manifest in skin at a later time during the course of disease. An alternative explanation would be the earlier possibility of diagnosis in the eye because of much better optical properties of the structures to be examined. Fluorescence video microscopy of the skin has to be carried out through the intact skin of humans with relatively poor transparency.

There is an interesting parallel between retina/vitreous and skin. Evidence has been produced that the main membrane restricting NaF diffusion in the eye is retinal pigmented epithelium and not the wall of retinal capillaries (28, 54). In nailfold capillaries, the capillary wall and in particular the outer border of the halo are less efficient diffusion barriers in diabetics than in normals. Whereas the reversibility of NaF penetration into the vitreous has been demonstrated under rigorous metabolic control (50), no such data are yet available for human skin.

At present, there is no capillaroscopic method to demonstrate the increased permeability of microvessels to macromolecules as shown by isotopes (16, 34). The ICG technique is probably not sensitive enough to assess protein transport through the wall of microvessels. In alloxan-treated Syrian hamsters, preferential sites of increased leakage of fluorescent macromolecules are located in small venules (8, 22).

Apart from symmetrically enhanced diffusion out of capillary loops, there is also experimental evidence that newly formed vessels exhibit particularly increased permeability (26).

There is increasing experimental evidence (19, 52, 53, 54) that pharmacologic agents like sorbinil or aldose reductase inhibitors at least partially prevent damage to microvessels by blocking the altered biochemical pathways. Prospective clinical trials will have to prove whether these drugs are useful for the secondary prophylaxis of diabetic microangiopathy.

Microvascular Aspects of the "Diabetic Foot"

The swollen foot with incipient gangrene threatening limb survival is one of the major complications of diabetes. Unlike in gangrene without metabolic disease, foot pulses are often palpable. Neuropathy and infection are involved in the pathogenesis of the condition. The contribution of microangiopathy, however, remains controversial.

Even with palpable pulses *macroangiopathy* is not ruled out. Stenoses of proximal arteries, like the superficial femoral, may only dampen distal pulses. Calf arteries are very often involved. If two of them are occluded, pulse wave transmission through the third major channel may be sufficient to allow pulses to be palpable. Careful investigation for macroangiopathy, including arteriography and/or duplex scanning, is mandatory in every instance of a diabetic foot.

Neuropathy complicates the situation by rendering gangrene less painful and by favoring the development of skin lesions. Neuropathy contributes to the diabetic foot not only by decreasing skin sensibility, but also by impairing vasomotor reflexes (14, 15, 43). Malum perforans located at the sole is mostly caused by neuropathy, skin lesions at the tip of toes and at the lateral aspect of the foot by angiopathy. At the heel, the genesis of ulcers is mostly multifactorial (compression during bed rest, neuropathy, angiopathy).

Diabetics are more prone to *infections* than nondiabetics. Infection may involve the subcutaneous tissue, joints, or bones. Depending on the given clinical situation, infection plays a major or minor role in the pathogenesis of the diabetic foot.

In a review (31) it has been pointed out that there is no proof for the participation of diabetic *microangiopathy* in the clinical picture of the diabetic foot. Indeed, occlusive lesions of arterioles are as common in atherosclerotic disease without diabetes as with diabetes (9). In both conditions obstructions of arterioles abound. These changes are probably responsible for the fact that gangrene often concerns single toes or limited areas of the foot. In these regions threatened by necrosis, the number of blood-filled capillaries is drastically reduced (13).

On the other hand, *functional* abnormalities at the microvascular level should be considered as possible contributing factors. Altered microvascular hemodynamics and increased permeability, as described in this chapter, are the most likely candidates. Microangiopathy may favor the development of edema in the absence of infection or aggravate inflammatory edema. The diabetic foot results mostly from a combination of macroangiopathy, neuropathy, infection, and functional microangiopathy.

References 2.2

1) Ajjam, Z. S., Barton, S., Corbett, M., Owens, D., Marks, R.: Quantitative evaluation of the dermal vasculature of diabetics. *Quart. J. Med.* 215, 229–239, 1985.
2) Alpert, J. S., Coffman, J. D., Balodimos, M. C., Koncz, L., Soeldner, J. S.: Capillary permeability and blood flow in skeletal muscle of patients with diabetes mellitus and genetic prediabetes. *N. Engl. J. Med.* 286, 454–460, 1972.
3) Bollinger, A., Frey, J., Jäger, K., Furrer, J., Seglias, J., Siegenthaler, W.: Patterns of diffusion through skin capillaries in patients with long-term diabetes. *N. Engl. J. Med.* 307, 1305–1310, 1982.
4) Boulton, A. M. J., Scarpello, J. H. B., Ward, J. D.: Venous oxygen in the diabetic neuropathic foot. Evidence of arterio-venous shunting? *Diabetologia* 22, 6–8, 1982.
5) Brownlee, J., Cerami, A., Vlassara, H.: Advanced glycosylation end products in tissue and the biochemical basis of diabetic complications. *N. Engl. J. Med.* 318, 1315–1321, 1988.
6) Chazan, B. I., Balodimos, M. C., Lavine, R. L., Koncz, L.: Capillaries of the nailfold of the toe in diabetes mellitus. *Microvasc. Res.* 2, 504–507, 1970.
7) Coget, J. M., Dupuis-Uvny, Ch., Merlen, J. F.: Intérêt de l'étude de la conjonctive oculaire dans le dépistage du prédiabète. *J. Malad. Vasc.* 14, 68–70, 1989.
8) Colantuoni, A., Cimini, V., Coppini, G., Bertuglia, S.: Functional microangiopathy in alloxan-treated Syrian hamsters. *Int. J. Microcirc.: Clin. Exp.* 7, 105–122, 1988.
9) Conrad, M. C.: Abnormalities of the digital vasculature as related to ulceration and gangrene. *Circulation* 38, 568–580, 1968.
10) Cunha-Vaz, J. G., Gray, J. R., Zeimer, C., Mota, C., Ishimoto, B. M., Leite, E.: Characterization of the early stages of diabetic retinopathy by vitreous fluorophotometry. *Diabetes* 34, 53–59, 1985.
11) Dahl-Jörgensen, K., Brinchmann-Hansen, O., Hanssen, K. F., Ganes, T., Kierulf, P., Smeland, E., Sandvik, L., Aagenaes, O.: Ef-

fect of near normoglycaemia for two years on progression of early diabetic retinopathy, nephropathy and neuropathy: The Oslo Study. *Br. Med. J.* 293, 1195–1199, 1986.
12) Ditzel, J., Duckers, J.: The bulbar conjunctival vascular bed in diabetic children. *Acta Paed. Scand.* 46, 535–552, 1957.
13) Fagrell, B., Hermansson, I. -L., Karlander, S. -G., Östergren, J.: Vital capillary microscopy for assessment of skin viability and microangiopathy in patients with diabetes mellitus. *Acta Med. Scand.* Suppl. 687, 25–28, 1984.
14) Farris, I., Nielsen, H. V., Henriksen, O., Parving, H. -H., Lassen, N. A.: Impaired autoregulation of blood flow in skeletal muscle and subcutaneous tissue in long-term type I (insulin-dependent) diabetic patients with microangiopathy. *Diabetologia* 25, 486–488, 1983.
15) Farris, I., Duncan, H.: Vascular disease and vascular function in the lower limb in diabetes. *Diabet. Res.* 1, 171–177, 1984.
16) Feldt-Rasmussen, B.: Increased transcapillary escape rate of albumin in type I (insulin-dependent) diabetic patients with microalbuminuria. *Diabetologia* 29, 282–286, 1986.
17) Fenton, B. M., Zweifach, B. W., Worthen, D. M.: Quantitative morphometry of conjunctival microcirculation in diabetes mellitus. *Microvasc. Res.* 18, 153–166, 1979.
18) Frey, J., Furrer, J., Bollinger, A.: Transkapillare Diffusion von Na-Fluoreszein in Hautarealen des Fußrückens bei juvenilen Diabetikern. *Schweiz. med. Wschr.* 113, 1964–1969, 1983.
19) Greene, D. A., Lattimer, S. A., Sima, A. A. F.: Sorbitol, phosphoinositides and sodium-potassium-ATPase in the pathogenesis of diabetic complications. *N. Engl. J. Med.* 316, 599–606, 1987.
20) Jörneskog, G., Östergren, J., Tydén, G., Bolinder, J., Fagrell, B.: Is skin microvascular reactivity improved in diabetics after pancreas and kidney transplantation? *Int. J. Microcirc.: Clin. Exp.* 6, 186, 1987.
21) Jörneskog, G., Östergren, J., Fagrell, B., Tydén, G., Bolinder, J.: *Skin microvascular reactivity in type 1 diabetics with severe microangiopathy: The influence of kidney transplantation.* 1st Mediterranean Congress of Angiology, May 29–June 3, Corfu, Greece, 1988. (abstract)
22) Joyner, W. L., Mayhan, W. G., Johnson, R. L., Phares, C. K.: Microvascular alterations developed in Syrian hamsters after the induction of diabetes mellitus by streptozotocin. *Diabetes* 30, 93–100, 1981.
23) Jünger, M., Frey-Schnewlin, G., Bollinger, A.: Microvascular flow distribution and transcapillary diffusion at the forefoot in patients with peripheral ischemia. *Int. J. Microcirc.: Clin. Exp.* 8, 3–24, 1989.
24) Kastrup, J., Norgaard, T., Parving, H. -H., Henriksen, O., Lassen, N. A.: Impaired autoregulation of blood flow in subcutaneous tissue of long-term type I (insulin-dependent) diabetic patients with microangiopathy: An index of arteriolar dysfunction. *Diabetologia* 28, 711–717, 1985.
25) Katz, M. A., McNeill, G.: Defective vasodilation response to exercise in cutaneous precapillary vessels in diabetic humans. *Diabetes* 36, 1386–1396, 1987.
26) Kilzer, P., Chang, K., Marvel, J., Rowold, E., Jaudes, P., Ullensvang, S., Kilo, Ch., Williamson, J. R.: Albumin permeation of new vessels is increased in diabetic rats. *Diabetes* 34, 333–336, 1985.
27) Kjaergaard, J. J., Dideriksen, K., Mourits-Anderson, T.: Some aspects of the pharmacokinetics of fluorescein in normal and in diabetic subjects. *Int. J. Microcirc.: Clin. Exp.* 2, 191–197, 1983.
28) Krupin, R., Waltman, S. R.: Fluorometry in juvenile-onset diabetes, long-term follow-up. *Jpn. J. Ophtalmol.* 29, 139–145, 1985.
29) Lauritzen, T., Frost-Larsen, K., Larsen, H. W., Deckert, T.: Steno Study Group. Two year experience with continuous subcutaneous insulin infusion in relation to retinopathy and neuropathy. *Diabetes* 35, 74–79, 1985.
30) Leinonen, H., Matikainen, E., Juntunen, J.: Permeability and morphology of skeletal muscle capillaries in type I (insulin-dependent) diabetes mellitus. *Diabetologia* 22, 158–162, 1982.
31) Lo Gerfo, F. W., Coffman, J. D.: Vascular

and microvascular disease of the foot in diabetes. *N. Engl. J. Med.* 311, 1615–1619, 1984.

32) Mahler, F., Fuchs, Ch., Zürcher, S.: Nailfold capillary loop enlargement in diabetic patients. In Tsuchiya, M., Asano, M., Mishima, Y., Oda, M. (eds.)., *Microcirculation, an update*. Excerpta med., Amsterdam, New York, Oxford, 599–604, 1987.

33) McMillan, D. E., Haley, J. A.: The microcirculation: Changes in diabetes mellitus. *Mayo Clin. Proc.* 63, 517–520, 1988.

34) Parving, H. -H., Rossing, N.: Simultaneous determination of the transcapillary escape rate of albumin and IgG in the normal and long-term juvenile diabetic subjects. *Scand. J. Clin. Lab. Invest.* 32, 239–244, 1973.

35) Parving, H. -H., Hommel, E., Mathiesen, E., Skott, P., Edsberg, B., Bahnsen, M., Lauritzen, M., Hougaard, Ph.: Prevalence of microalbuminuria, arterial hypertension, retinopathy and neuropathy in patients with insulin dependent diabetes. *Brit. Med. J.* 296, 156–160, 1988.

36) Porta, M., La Selva, M., Molinatti, P., Molinatti, G. M.: Endothelial cell function in diabetic microangiopathy. *Diabetologia* 30, 601–609, 1987.

37) Rouen, L. R., Terry, E. N., Doft, B. H., Clauss, R. H., Redisch, W.: Classification and measurement of surface microvessels in man. *Microvasc. Res.* 4, 285–292, 1972.

38) Thüring-Vollenweider, U., Zimmermann, D., Moneta, G., Schnewlin, G., Froesch, E. R., Bollinger, A.: The influence of varying disease duration on transcapillary diffusion of sodium-fluorescein in forefoot skin of type I diabetics. In preparation.

39) Tilton, R. G., Faller, A. M., Burkhardt, J. K., Hoffmann, P. L., Kilo, C., Williamson, J. R.: Pericyte degeneration and acellular capillaries are increased in the feet of human diabetic patients. *Diabetologia* 28, 895–900, 1985.

40) Tooke, J. E.: A capillary pressure disturbance in young diabetics. *Diabetes*, 29, 815–819, 1980.

41) Tooke, J. E., Lins, P. E., Östergren, J., Adamson, U., Fagrell, B.: The effects of intravenous insulin infusion on skin microcirculatory flow in Type 1 diabetes. *Int. J. Microcirc.: Clin.Exp.* 4, 63–68, 1985.

42) Tooke, J. E., Lins, P. -E., Östergren, J., Fagrell, B.: Skin microvascular autoregulatory responses in type I diabetes: the influence of duration and control. *Int. J. Microcirc.: Clin. Exp.* 4, 249–256, 1985.

43) Tooke, J. E.: Microvascular haemodynamics in diabetes mellitus. *Clin. Sci.* 70, 119–125, 1986.

44) Tooke, J. E.: Nailfold capillary pressure measurement. *Prog. appl. Microcirc.* 11, 60–73, 1986

45) Tooke, J. E., Östergren, J., Lins, P. E., Fagrell, B.: Skin microvascular blood flow control in long duration diabetics with and without complications. *Diabetes Research* 5, 189–192, 1987.

46) Tooke, J. E.: Microcirculation and diabetes. *Brit. Med. Bull.* 45, 206–223, 1989.

47) Trap-Jensen, J.: Increased permeability to ^{131}iodide and (^{51}CR) EDTA in the exercising forearm of long-term diabetics. *Clin. Sci.* 39, 39–49, 1970.

48) Tymms, D. J., Tooke, J. E.: The effect of continuous subcutaneous insulin infusion (CSII) on microvascular blood flow in diabetes mellitus. *Int. J. Microcirc.: Clin. Exp.* 7, 347–356, 1988.

49) Vermes, I., Steinmetz, E. T., Zeyen, L. J. J. M., van der Veen, E. A.: Rheological properties of white blood cells are changed in diabetic patients with microvascular complications. *Diabetologia* 30, 434–436, 1987.

50) White, N. H., Waltman, S. R., Krupin, T., Santiago, J. V.: Reversal of abnormalities in ocular fluorophotometry in insulin-dependent diabetes after five to nine months of improved metabolic control. *Diabetes* 31, 80–85, 1982.

51) Williamson, J. R., Kilo, C.: Current status of capillary basement-membrane disease in diabetes mellitus. *Diabetes* 26, 65–73, 1977.

52) Williamson, J. R., Chang, K., Rowold, E., Marvel, J., Tomlinson, M., Sherman, W. R., Ackermann, K. E., Kilo, C.: Sorbinil prevents diabetes-induced increases in vascular permeability but does not alter collagen cross-linking. *Diabetes* 34, 703–705, 1985.

53) Williamson, J. R., Rowold, E., Chang, K.:

Sex steroid dependency of diabetes-induced changes in polyol metabolism, vascular permeability, and collagen cross-linking. *Diabetes* 35, 20–27, 1986.

54) Winegrad, A. I.: Does a common mechanism induce the diverse complications of diabetes? *Diabetes* 36, 396–406, 1987.

55) Yanko, L., Davis, E.: Conjunctival microangiopathy in diabetic retinopathy. *Microcirc.* 1, 55–68, 1981.

2.3 Chronic Venous Incompetence (CVI)

Chronic venous incompetence is caused either by postthrombotic changes of deep, perforator, and superficial veins of the lower extremities, or by primary varicous veins involving perforating and superficial veins. More or less marked deep valvular insufficiency may also be observed with primary varicous veins.

The main pathophysiologic factor responsible for the clinical features such as cyanosis, edema, hyperpigmentation, skin induration and white atrophy is sustained venous hypertension. Whereas in normal limbs exercise reduces venous pressure through the activation of the muscle pump for considerable periods of time, the pressure drop lasts briefly or is even abolished in CVI. Valvular insufficiency of deep and perforating veins prevents the muscle pump from working efficiently. Venous pressure increases during walking, with pressure heads in insufficient perforator veins elicited by each muscular contraction. Contributing factors include residual obstruction or only partial recanalization of thrombosed deep veins, valvular insufficiency of superficial veins, ankylosis of the ankle-joint, and paresis or paralysis of leg muscles impairing muscle pump.

These changes of venous macrocirculation induce important microvascular alterations that are probably the ultimate cause of trophic skin changes and ulcer development. Both blood and lymphatic capillaries participate in what has been called microangiopathy from CVI.

Changes of Capillary Morphology

Already in 1949 Gilje (15) showed that the skin microcirculation of the lower leg was considerably affected in patients with different stages of peripheral venous insufficiency. Later, Ryan (27) and Fagrell (12, 13) confirmed that the morphology of the skin capillaries changes dramatically in patients with venous insufficiency. However, it must be realized that microangiopathy from CVI shows a patchy distribution. In one particular skin region, for the most part close to the major insufficient perforators, severe changes may be present, whereas not far away only mild alterations or even normal skin capillaries may be found. The severe changes observed by clinical investigation are most often a reliable guide for the presence of microangiopathy, but sometimes it may be difficult to observe the pattern of capillary changes, for example, in areas with marked pigmentation or edema.

Superficial Venous Insufficiency

When only the *superficial venous system* is insufficient, the changes of the skin capillaries are

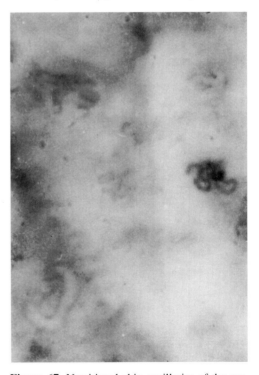

Figure 67. Nutritional skin capillaries of the medial side of the lower leg of a patient with mild deep venous insufficiency. The capillaries are dilated and tortuous.

moderate. They become coiled and distended (**Figure 67**). More severe changes are not present even in patients with marked superficial varicoses. The reason for this is most probably that the venous pressure in these patients is not markedly elevated, and accordingly the disturbance of the skin circulation is limited (1).

Deep Venous Insufficiency (DVI) and/or Incompetent Perforators (IP)

The venous pressure in the lower leg of patients with DVI is not significantly elevated at rest in the sitting or standing position (1). However, during walking the pressure in the subcutaneous veins of the lower leg increases considerably, which produces a rapid and marked pressure increase in the microvascular bed of the skin in the affected region (1, 12, 13). This high pressure induces a capillary dilatation, and they become tortuous (**Figure 68**). The number of the capillaries per mm^2 is also reduced. Sometimes the capillaries look like glomeruli. A striking finding in most patients with DVI is a halo formation seen around the dilated capillaries. The halo in itself is caused by a very specific microedema in the skin papillae, which is not seen in any other patients with edema formation. The edema, which contains fibrin, proteins, and neutral polysaccharides (7, 8, 23), is

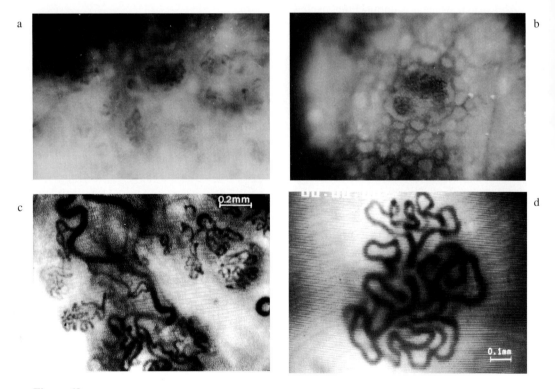

Figure 68.
a) Glomerulus-like capillaries with diffuse light areas surrounding the capillaries. This is a specific, papillary microedema seen only in patients with deep venous insufficiency (DVI).
b) A patient with marked DVI. A clear edema formation around tortuous capillaries can be seen. The skin cells are forming a pigmented network around the small edema pools.
c) Enlarged and tortuous capillaries with an effluent venule near the medial ankle of a patient with severe chronic venous incompetence.
d) Glomerulus-like capillary convolute at the medial ankle of another patient with severe CVI.

most probably the main reason for the abolished nutrition in the affected skin. When the patients are in a horizontal position, the pressure in the edematous papillae often exceeds the intracapillary pressure, leading to a collapse of the capillaries and an impaired nutrition. In the upright position, the transmural pressure increases considerably, and the capillaries become filled with blood. Nevertheless, nutrition is still impaired because the edema blocks the normal nutritional pathways between the capillaries and the skin cells (**Figure 69**). Consequently, this edema is one of the main causes for the impaired nutrition leading to the development of skin necrosis and venous leg ulcers. It should also be stressed that edema is most probably not formed only by the increase in the capillary pressure, but also because of an impaired lymphatic drainage from the area (see page 101). Edema formation can be nicely documented by the fluorescent technique, which can also be used for studying the dynamics of the edema formation in different stages of venous incompetence.

If the edema is not treated properly, it may slowly be organized, and the skin is destroyed and successively converted into a fibrous tissue (23). If the venous insufficiency is correctly treated with effective compression bandages, the edema is reduced and the skin cells come in contact with the capillaries, leading to a normalized nutrition (**Figure 70**). This is probably the main reason why compression therapy is so effective for healing venous skin ulcers.

Morphologic Studies by Fluorescence Video Microscopy

The fluorochrome NaF enhances image contrast especially in skin sections with poor transparency, identifies nonperfused capillaries or areas, and depicts the pericapillary halos more accurately than conventional capillaroscopy. Morphometry of halos becomes possible. Because of bright background fluorescence after application of NaF, studies of red blood cell flow are easier.

Halo Diameters

Mean halo diameters, ranging between the largest and smallest individual halo and standard deviations, are plotted in **Table 17** (17, 30) for controls and patients with mild and severe CVI. The pericapillary halo at the supramalleolar region is of circular shape. In normal controls individual halo limits are clearly separated from the neighboring halos (**Figure 71**). Normal halo diameter averages 81 ± 15 μm (14) at the medial ankle.

In both mild (30) and severe CVI (17), halo size is significantly (p<0.001) enhanced. In the latter condition mean halo size reached 146 ± 47 μm. The values indicated in **Table 17** are similar to the ones determined by Saner and

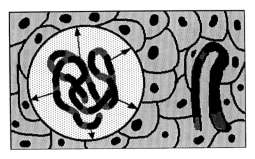

Figure 69. Schematic presentation of the specific microedema formation in patients with DVI. The edema presses the skin cells away, and blocks the pathway of nutrients from the capillaries to the cells. In normal subjects (right part of the picture), the skin cells are in intimate contact with the capillary.

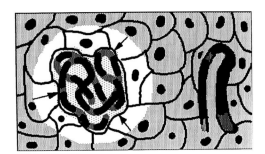

Figure 70. After compression therapy and/or diuretics, the microedema is diminished with an improved nutrition in the area.

coworkers (28) who performed the first morphometric study of halos in CVI. The distance between individual halos is reduced. The halo limits almost touch each other. The video microscopic image resembles a street covered with cobblestones, as is easily recognized in **Figure 71**.

In CVI, not only the absolute values of halo size are increased, but also the ranges between the smallest and largest halo observed in one individual patient (**Table 17**). Inhomogeneity of halo size is significantly ($p<0.05$) lower in patients with mild than with severe disease. This finding reflects increasing inhomogeneity during disease progression.

Whereas the halo diameters measured in healthy volunteers follow a Gaussian distribution, inhomogeneous distribution is typical in patients (**Figure 72**). Halos with normal and enlarged size coexist. In severe CVI, giant halos (>500 μm) containing extremely coiled and enlarged capillaries may be encountered (**Figure 73**). The red blood cells travel through the tortuous pathways like in a luna park.

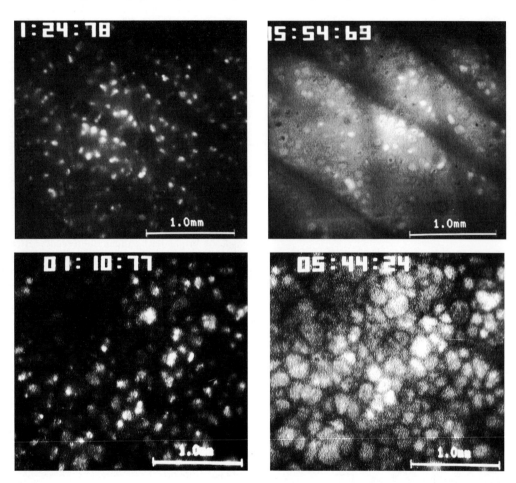

Figure 71.
Above: Images of a normal subject at the ankle about 1 and 15 min after NaF appearance. Small and regular pericapillary halos with large interhalo distances are filled.
Below: Corresponding pictures of a patient with moderate CVI. The halos are enlarged and of varying size. They almost touch each other ("cobblestone aspect").

Chronic Venous Incompetence (CVI)

Microvascular Thrombosis and White Cell Trapping

In a study dedicated to severe CVI (17), some giant and tortuous capillaries densely packed with erythrocytes did not show corpuscular flow and were not filled by NaF during almost an hour (**Figure 74**). Similar images have been observed in two other patients. This finding probably corresponds to microvascular thrombosis. The only alternative explanation is prolonged stasis of red blood cell aggregates in the enlarged and tortuous capillary loops.

Figure 72. Distribution of halo diameters in controls, patients with mild and severe CVI. n = number of measurements. The Gaussian distribution in normals is abolished in patients.

Table 17. Mean halo diameters, standard deviations and mean ranges of halo diameters in normal controls, patients with mild and severe chronic venous incompetence (µm) according to Haselbach et al. (17), Speiser and Bollinger (30).

	Diameter	Range
Controls (n = 8)	81±15 (28–134)	106±26
Mild CVI (n = 8)	138±41* (58–219)	161±54*
Severe CVI (n = 10)	146±47*	245±87** (24–629)

* significant difference to controls ($p < 0.001$)
** significant difference to controls ($p<0.001$) and to patients with mild CVI ($p<0.05$)

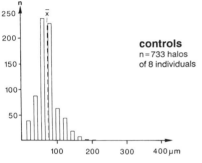

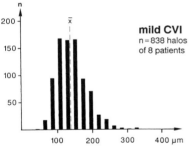

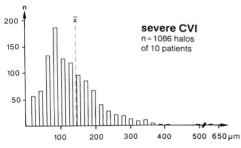

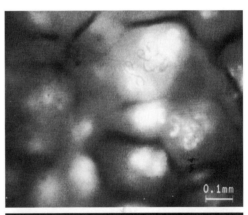

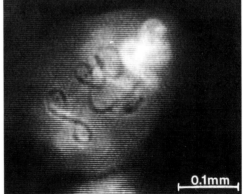

Figure 73.
Above: Enlarged pericapillary halos stained by NaF containing meandering capillaries.
Below: Larger magnification of a glomerulus-like convolute with surrounding pericapillary halo.

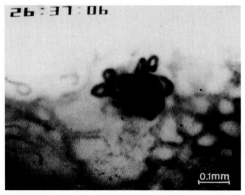

Figure 74. Glomerulus-like capillary convolute with densely packed red blood cells not yet perfused by NaF 26 min 37 s after dye injection. The bright background results from the fluorescent tracer delivered by adjacent perfused microvessels. The image probably corresponds to capillary thrombosis.

Table 18. Mean fluorescent light intensities and standard errors in percent of the individual intensity at different times from first dye appearance in a rectangular area above the medial ankle encompassing 3.2 mm^2 (17, 30). Capillary density is given in numbers per mm^2.

	Controls (n = 15)	Mild CVI (n = 15)	Severe CVI (n = 15)
5 s	3.6±0.7	9.7±2.1*	3.7± 3.5
10 s	5.9±1.3	13.0±2.5*	10.2±12.3
30 s	14.7±2.3	24.1±3.4*	20.6±16.9
60 s	23.6±2.9	31.4±3.3*	26.8±14.9
2 min	36.9±3.6	44.6±2.6*	39.3±13.1
5 min	62.6±3.6	73.9±2.7*	67.6±11.5
10 min	86.6±2.8	94.5±1.5*	89.8± 5.7
20 min	96.8±1.1	91.5±2.5	93.4± 7.9
capillary	27.0±6.9°	26.3±6.8°	24.4± 6.1°
density	41.4±7.2°°	41.5±6.4°°	41.6± 8.3°°

° 1 minute after dye arrival; °° 5 minutes after dye arrival
* significant differences (p<0.05) compared to the control group

Histological studies prove that microvascular thrombosis may develop in severe CVI (29, 32). Moreover, the presence of *atrophie blanche* in many patients (3, 4) corroborates the existence of microvascular thrombosis, since the formation of avascular fields is difficult to explain by alternative mechanisms. Definite intravital microscopic evidence could only be gained by serial examinations demonstrating the disappearance of loops previously filled by stagnant red blood cells.

A supplementary or alternative explanation for microvascular occlusion is white cell trapping in microvessels (10, 31). It has been shown that 28.6% of the white blood cells accumulate in sitting position in the leg of patients with severe CVI, but only 5% in healthy controls (p<0.01). Moreover, hemoconcentration with dependent legs is more pronounced in patients than in healthy volunteers (31). Although most of the white cells are washed out when resuming a supine position, repeated trapping could damage the capillary wall, increase permeability, and predispose to microthrombosis. There is also evidence that the number of skin capillaries perfused by erythrocytes decreases in sitting patients compared to controls (31), which has been explained by temporal blocking of loops by white cells.

Transcapillary and Interstitial Diffusion of NaF

Skin Areas

Fluorescence video microscopy in combination with densitometry has been applied to 15 healthy controls, 15 patients with mild CVI, and 15 patients with severe CVI (17, 30). The patients with minor disease complained of swelling and heavy legs and had slight oedema corona phlebectatica and cyanosis in the upright position (stage I according to Widmer [33]). Skin induration, hyperpigmentation, or healed ulcers were present in the group with pronounced CVI (stages II or III).

Transcapillary diffusion was determined in a skin area of 3.2 mm^2 just above the medial ankle. The values for the three groups are given in **Table 18**. In the patients with severe CVI, care was taken to exclude skin regions with an apparently decreased number of capillary loops. Mean fluorescent light intensity was significantly ($p<0.05$) enhanced in the group with mild CVI only. Although the values in severe CVI tended to be higher than in the normal controls, the difference did not reach statistical significance.

There are different possible reasons for the unexpected difference between mild and severe disease. Burnand et al. (8) and Wenner et al. (32) have shown that pericapillary fibrin layers encircle the capillaries in CVI. The deposition of these macromolecules could influence the diffusion of small solutes like NaF into the interstitial space. It is possibly more pronounced in severe than in mild disease. Other potential factors reducing transcapillary diffusion in severe CVI compared to moderate disease include asynchronous inflow of the dye, which has been detected in several cases with severe, but in none with mild CVI; and microvascular obliterations by thrombosis or stable red blood cell aggregates decreasing the surface area available for diffusion. Moreover, lymphatic microangiopathy described below is absent or minor in mild CVI. In severe CVI the superficial network of lymphatic capillaries is interrupted by obliterations or even destroyed completely (5, 19). Impaired lymphatic drainage may alter the composition of interstitial fluid and proteins and elevate interstitial pressure possibly diminishing transcapillary diffusion of NaF. White cell trapping, which is supposed to modify capillary permeability (10, 31), might also be lower in the very large meandering capillaries more common in severe disease.

That there was no significant increase of transcapillary diffusion in skin areas of patients with severe CVI (17) does not exclude enhanced leakage of small and large molecules into single pericapillary halos containing enlarged and coiled capillaries. Transcapillary diffusion has not been evaluated at the single capillary level, but Fagrell (12) has punctured halos with increased size that partially collapsed after evacuation of edema fluid. Border capillaries of avascular fields of *atrophie blanche* exhibit increased transcapillary diffusion compared to loops away from the border (4). Work with the suction blister technique (2) showed increased permeability in mild and severe CVI, probably because of mechanical halo damage and evacuation.

As mentioned, microangiopathy in CVI is distributed in a patchy way. Severe microvascular lesions may be found next to vessels with minor changes. This should be taken into account whenever microvascular studies are planned in patients with CVI. Rarefaction of capillary loops is of particular importance (4, 14). A direct relationship between reduced capillary number and decreased transcutaneous oxygen tension was established (14). In regions devoid of capillaries, oxygen delivery to the skin surface may be close to zero. Mild CVI is characterized by normal or subnormal transcutaneous oxygen tension, severe CVI in regions with decreased number of perfused capillaries by microvascular ischemia (6, 9, 14, 20, 22, 24). These findings concerning the nutritional capillaries of the skin do not contradict the finding that increased flow is measured by positron emission tomography in the subcutis (16), where arterio-venous anastomoses are present.

White Atrophy (Atrophie Blanche)

Development of *atrophie blanche* is not limited to CVI. Typical lesions are also observed in progressive systemic sclerosis (see page 123) and other forms of collagen vascular disease. Earlier workers considered white atrophy to be an independent entity or attributed it to various clinical conditions including syphilis. Today, it appears that *atrophie blanche* is a lesion indicating microvascular disease of different etiology. It may be interpreted as small cutaneous infarction resulting from obliteration of larger microvessels and capillaries (3, 29).

Intravital anatomy of *atrophie blanche* due to CVI and diffusion of NaF into the avascular field were studied in 12 patients (4). The lesions were located near the medial ankle. Mean diameter of white atrophy was about 1 mm.

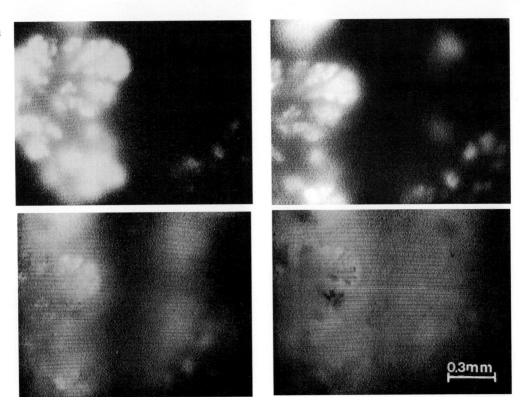

H. M. ♀, 48y.

Figure 75.
a) Fluorescence video microscopy with NaF over a field of *atrophie blanche* (patient with severe CVI) 30 s, 2 min 30 s, 10 min, and 20 min after NaF appearance on the lower leg. First, the ramified border capillaries fluoresce; then, the dye diffuses toward the center of the dark avascular field, which slowly becomes brighter.
b) Three-dimensional analysis of fluorescent light intensity in another patient with white atrophy measured by video densitometry on an axis crossing the field.
below a and c: border capillaries on each side; b: center of the area devoid of microvessels. The "valley" pattern (peak intensity over border capillaries) is typical for early times after NaF appearance, the "mountain" pattern for the late times when peak intensity is recorded from the center.

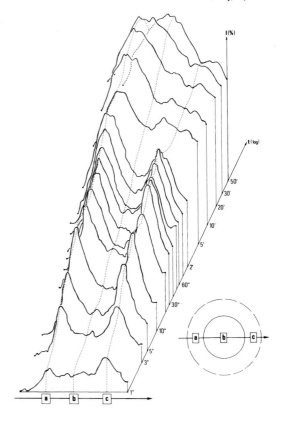

Chronic Venous Incompetence (CVI)

Intravital Anatomy

Spots of white atrophy can be recognized by the naked eye and may exceptionally reach diameters of several millimeters or even centimeters. They are mostly localized around the medial ankle. Intravital microscopy reveals three main areas:

- the avascular field sensu strictu with no recognizable capillaries,
- the enlarged and meandering capillaries at the edge of the lesion lying approximately parallel to the skin surface,
- the remote area with more or less altered capillaries emerging from below.

An example is given in **Figure 75**. The diameter of the border capillaries averages 30–40 µm. In many of the larger lesions not included in this study, megacapillaries or capillary convolutes emerge as islets from deeper skin layers. They appear as dots within the avascular area.

Transcapillary and Interstitial Diffusion

The different steps of NaF diffusion into the avascular field are illustrated by **Figure 75**. Measurements of fluorescent light intensity on an axis crossing the field at different times document the pattern of interstitial diffusion (**Figure 75**). Promptly after reaching the loops, the dye leaves the intravascular compartment and moves slowly toward the center of the avascular region. At early times the tracings assume a "valley-like" aspect with peaks of high fluorescent light intensity over the border capillaries and lower intensity over the capillaries away from the border. Interstitial diffusion to the avascular center takes as long as 20–40 minutes. At these late times, peak light intensity is located at the central areas since the "valley" has been slowly filled up by the dye and fluorescence faded over the border capillaries (**Figure 75**). In normal ankle skin, fluorescent light intensity is distributed homogeneously and does not show "valley" formation at video densitometry (4). Densitometer curves along an axis crossing a number of normal loops are horizontal at any time after dye appearance.

When fluorescent light intensity over the three characteristic zones is plotted against time, the peak values are significantly higher over the border capillaries than over the capillaries away from the border ($p<0.05$–0.001). This finding may be explained by increased transcapillary diffusion, but as well, at least in part, by enhanced surface area available for diffusion in the enlarged and tortuous border capillaries. Maximal fluorescent light intensity at the avascular center of the field is reached when the values already drop in the perfused regions. Only after 20 minutes does the concentration gradient between the border and the center of the field reverse, marking the begin of dye clearance out of the *atrophie blanche* spot.

The turnover of substances involved in tissue nutrition is probably as slow as demonstrated for NaF. The clinical experience that skin regions containing fields of white atrophy are predilection sites for ulcer formation is explained by these dynamic studies of diffusion. This view is supported by transcutaneous oxygen tension measurements which revealed values close to zero in fields of *atrophie blanche* (14).

Lymphatic Microangiopathy

Fluorescence microlymphography (5) and indirect lymphography with water-soluble contrast media (25) opened up new ways to study lymphatic microcirculation in CVI. It was earlier demonstrated that micromolecules labeled by radioisotopes are drained to a lesser extent when they are injected into dermatosclerotic areas than into the intact skin of the foot dorsum (21).

After subepidermal injection of FITC-dextran 150,000 (see page 54) the *lymphatic capillaries* or initial lymphatics fill from the dye deposit. No marked changes of capillary morphology are observed in patients without trophic skin changes (5). The propagation of the dye into the superficial network is increased, however.

It is probable that lymphatic vessels transport at least a part of the increased volume of tissue fluid during early CVI. There is ample experimental evidence that venous obstruction induces an increase in net filtration which expands interstitial volume and enhances lymph flow (11, 26).

Definite microangiopathy is found in skin areas of the medial ankle presenting with induration and hyperpigmentation (5, 19). Some meshes of the network are interrupted by obliterations (**Figure 76**). Fragments of capillaries may be stained quite far away from the dye deposit. Precollectors and collectors opacified by water-soluble contrast media are dilated and of irregular shape (25). It has been postulated that these changes result from long-lasting overcharges of draining microlymphatics which remove increased amounts of interstitial fluid.

As in mild CVI, dye expansion into the superficial network is enhanced (see **Figure 85**, page 111), probably because of impeded drainage into the deeper precollectors and collectors. Mean maximal propagation from the border of the dye depot into one of the four directions reached 7.8 ± 2.6 mm in normals and 25.4 ± 21.6 mm in patients with CVI (p<0.005).

In extreme cases, no lymphatic capillaries are filled at all, even when several depots of FITC-dextran 150,000 are placed. The dye

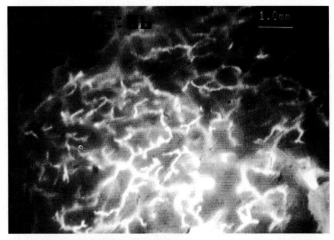

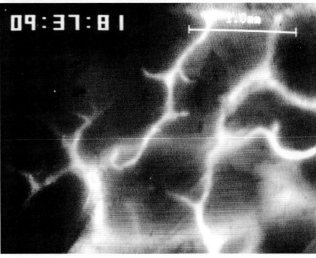

Figure 76.
Above: Lymphatic microangiopathy in a patient with severe CVI near the medial ankle. The network is interrupted by multiple obliterations.
Below: Obliterations of lymphatic capillaries at a larger magnification.

Chronic Venous Incompetence (CVI)

General Concept

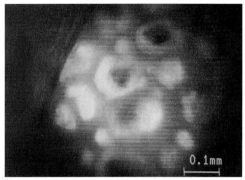

Figure 77. Cutaneous reflux of fluorescent material far away from the depot of FITC-dextran 150,000. Most intensive fluorescence is located around dark blood capillaries appearing as dots. Prelymphatic pathways probably run close to the superficial loops.

As outlined, changes of venous macrocirculatory dynamics, especially valvular incompetence, induce progressive damage to blood microvessels. The capillaries dilate, elongate, and coil. They are embedded in pericapillary halos of increased size containing edema fluid. Transcapillary diffusion in skin areas is enhanced. Lymphatic capillary morphology remains intact in early stages. Probably, the increased amount of fluid and macromolecules accumulated in the

propagates into the interstitial space without clear-cut pathways (5).

Cutaneous reflux of FITC-dextran 150,000 occurs in some patients with CVI (5, 19). First, the dye moves into deeper, invisible structures and reappears at the visible surface away from the dye deposit. **Figure 77** shows a particularly interesting example for cutaneous reflux. The dye emerges from below not in lymphatic capillaries, but around dilated blood capillaries, suggesting that the pericapillary halo region is in direct retrograde communication with deeper channels. Valvular insufficiency and retrograde motion in precollectors and collectors is illustrated by water-soluble contrast media (25). Unlike in normals, dermal backflow depicts enlarged microvessels (**Figure 78**).

In healthy controls, the meshes of the superficial capillary network are well delineated up to one hour. No or only minor leakage of FITC dextran 150,000 is observed. In some patients with CVI, permeability of microlymphatics was increased (5). The fragmented network is clearly outlined for only 10–40 minutes after dye injection. Later the capillaries become blurred. Cloudy diffuse fluorescence appears where the capillaries had previously been visualized (**Figure 79**). The fluorescent macromolecules enter the damaged microvessels but leave them in part by leaking through the capillary wall: A vicious circle is created.

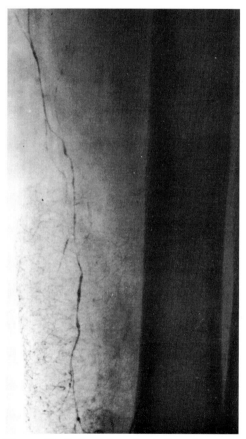

Figure 78. Indirect lymphography with water-soluble contrast medium in a patient with CVI (Prof. H. Partsch, Vienna). From the subepidermal pool, precollectors are opacified. Reflux of contrast medium from deeper channels to superficial skin through vessels with valvular insufficiency is evident.

Figure 79. Fluorescence microlymphography in a patient with severe CVI showing increased microvascular permeability.
Above: Irregular network of initial lymphatics interrupted by obliterations (4 min 18 s after injection of FITC-dextran 150,000).
Below: At 24 min 31 s, the lymphatic microvessels are no more delineated. The diffuse patchy fluorescence of the interstitial space originates from dye molecules that have permeated through the wall of damaged capillaries and regained the interstitial space.

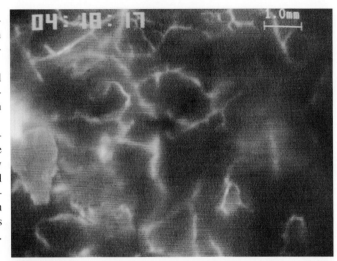

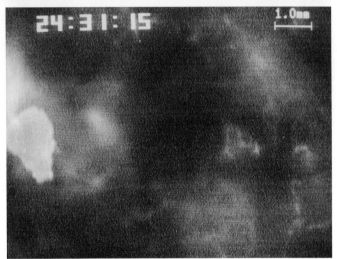

interstitial space is drained by compensatory augmentation of lymph flow.

With progression of disease, the microangiopathy of blood capillaries worsens. The number of capillaries decreases because of obliterations of microvessels that may be blocked by microvascular thrombosis (17) or trapped white blood cells (10, 31). Avascular areas develop. Although there are still microvessels with increased transcapillary diffusion, like the meandering border capillaries of *atrophie blanche*, transcapillary diffusion in skin areas is no longer significantly enhanced. On the other hand, lymphatic microangiopathy now contributes to edema formation. Macromolecules not only enter microlymphatics but also leak out of them in a vicious circle. Indurated edema and dermatosclerosis of skin are at least in part the result of lymphatic involvement that may be aggravated by recurrent infections.

Reduced capillary number, pathologic shape of remaining capillary loops within enlarged halos, and lymphatic microangiopathy create a situation in which tissue nutrition is jeopardized. Indeed, transcutaneous oxygen tension is low or extremely low in regions with most evident microvascular changes (14). Venous ulcers form in skin with microvascular ischemia and combined venous and lymphatic edema.

References 2.3

1) Arnoldi, C. C., Linderholm, H.: On the pathogenesis of the venous leg ulcer. *Acta. Chir. Scand.* 134, 427–440, 1968.
2) Belcaro, G., Rulo, A.: A study of capillary permeability in patients with venous hypertension by a new system: the vacuum suction chamber (VSG) device—A preliminary report. *Phlebology* 3, 255–259, 1988.
3) Bollinger, A.: Atrophie blanche: Hautinfarkt verschiedener Pathogenese? *VASA* 10, 67–69, 1981.
4) Bollinger, A.: Transcapillary and interstitial diffusion of Na-fluorescein in chronic venous insufficiency with white atrophy. *Int. J. Microcirc.: Clin. Exp.* 1, 5–17, 1982.
5) Bollinger, A., Isenring, G., Franzeck, U. K.: Lymphatic microangiopathy: a complication of severe chronic venous incompetence (CVI). *Lymphology* 15, 60–65, 1982.
6) Borzykowski, M., Krahenbuhl, B.: Mesure noninvasive de l'oxygénation cutanée chronique des membres inférieurs. *Schweiz. med. Wschr.* 111, 1972–1974, 1981.
7) Browse, N. L., Burnand, K. G.: The cause of venous ulceration. *Lancet* 2, 243–245, 1982.
8) Burnand, K. G., Whimster, I., Naidoo, A., Browse, N. L.: Pericapillary fibrin in the ulcer-bearing skin of the leg: The cause of lipodermatosclerosis and venous ulceration. *Brit. Med. J.* 285, 1071–1072, 1982.
9) Carpentier, P., Magne, J. L., Sarrot-Reynauld, F., Franco, A.: Insuffisance veineuse chronique et microcirculation. Réflexions physiopathologiques et thérapeutiques. *J. Malad. Vasc.* (Paris) 12, 280–284, 1987.
10) Coleridge Smith, P. D., Thomas, P., Scurr, J. H., Dormandy, J. A.: Causes of venous ulceration: A new hypothesis. *Brit. Med. J.* 296, 1726–1727, 1988.
11) Fadnes, H. O.: Effect of increased venous pressure on the hydrostatic and colloid osmotic pressure in subcutaneous interstitial fluid in rats: Edema preventing mechanisms. *Scand. J. Clin. Invest.* 36, 371–377, 1976.
12) Fagrell, B.: Local microcirculation in chronic venous incompetence and leg ulcers. *Vasc. Surg.* 13, 217–225, 1979.
13) Fagrell, B.: Microcirculatory disturbances—The final cause for venous leg ulcers? *VASA* 11, 101–103, 1982.
14) Franzeck, U. K., Bollinger, A., Huch, R., Huch, A.: Transcutaneous oxygen tension and capillary morphologic characteristics and density in patients with chronic venous incompetence. *Circulation* 70, 806–811, 1984.
15) Gilje, O.: Ulcus cruris in venous circulatory disturbances. *Acta Derm.-Venereol.* (Suppl. 22), 29, 1949.
16) Gowland Hopkins, N. F., Spinks, T. J., Rhodes, C. G., Ranicar, A. S. O., Jamieson, C. W.: Positron emission tomography in venous ulceration and liposclerosis: Study of regional tissue function. *Brit. Med. J.* 286, 333–336, 1983.
17) Haselbach, P., Vollenweider, U., Moneta, G., Bollinger, A.: Microangiopathy in severe chronic venous insufficiency evaluated by fluorescence video -microscopy. *Phlebology* 1, 159–169, 1986.
18) Hertlein, W.: Ein Beitrag zur Technik der Kapillarmikroskopie. *Zschr. angew. Bäder-Klimahk.* 6, 54–59, 1959.
19) Jäger, K., Isenring, G., Bollinger, A.: Fluorescence microlymphography in patients with lymphedema and chronic venous incompetence. *Inter. Angio.* 3, 129–136, 1983.
20) Kolari, P. J., Pekanmäki, K., Pohjola, R. T.: Transcutaneous oxygen tension in patients with post-thrombotic leg ulcers: Treatment with intermittent pneumatic compression. *Cardiovasc. Res.* 22, 138–141, 1988.
21) Lofferer, O., Mostbeck, A., Partsch, H.: Nuklearmedizinische Diagnostik von Lymphtransportstörungen der unteren Extremitäten. *VASA* 1, 94–102, 1972.
22) Mani, R., Gorman, F. W., White, J. E.: Transcutaneous measurements of oxygen tension at edges of leg ulcers: preliminary communication. *J. Roy. Soc. Med.* 79, 650–654, 1986.

23) Mani, R., White, J. E., Barett, D. F., Weaver, P. W.: Tissue oxygenation, venous ulcers and fibrin cuffs. *J. R. Soc. Med.* 82, 345, 1989.
24) Neumann, H. A. M., van Leeuwen, M., van den Broek, M. J. R. B., Berretty, P. J. M.: Transcutaneous oxygen tension in chronic venous insufficiency syndrome. *VASA* 13, 213–219, 1984.
25) Partsch, H., Urbanek, A., Wenzel-Hora, B.: Dermal lymphangiopathy in chronic venous incompetence. In Bollinger, A., Partsch, H., Wolfe, J. H. N. (eds.), *The initial lymphatics, new methods and findings*. Thieme, Stuttgart, New York, 178–187, 1985.
26) Renkin, E. M., Joyner, W. L., Sloop, C. H., Watson, P. D.: Influence of venous pressure on plasma-lymph transport in the dog's paw: convective and dissipative mechanisms. *Microvasc. Res.* 14, 191–204, 1977.
27) Ryan, T. J.: The epidermis and its blood supply in venous disorders of the leg. *Trans. St. John's Hosp. Derm. Soc.* (London) 55, 51, 1969.
28) Saner, H., Boss, Ch., Mahler, F.: Demonstration of the pericapillary space after intravenous administration of sodium fluorescein. In Bollinger, A., Partsch, H., Wolfe, J. H. N. (eds.), *The initial lymphatics, new methods and findings*. Thieme, Stuttgart, New York, 94–97, 1985.
29) Santler, R.: Atrophie blanche. *Hausarzt* 17, 346–348, 1966.
30) Speiser, D., Bollinger, A.: Microangiopathy in mild chronic venous incompetence. *Int. J. Microcirc.: Clin. Exp.* (in print).
31) Thomas, P. R. S., Nash, G. B., Dormandy, J. A.: White cell accumulation in dependent legs of patients with venous hypertension: a possible mechanism for trophic changes in the skin. *Brit. Med. J.* 296, 1693–1695, 1988.
32) Wenner, A., Leu, H. J., Spycher, M., Brunner, U.: Ultrastructural changes of capillaries in chronic venous insufficiency. *Expl. Cell Biol.* 48, 1–14, 1980.
33) Widmer, L. K., Stähelin, H. B., Nissen, C., Da Silva, A.: *Venen-, Arterienkrankheiten, koronare Herzkrankheit bei Berufstätigen. Prospektive epidemiologische Untersuchung. Basler Studie I–III 1958–1978.* Huber, Bern, 1981.

2.4 Lymphedema

Lymphedema was already a well-recognized entity in the last century. The extreme features of the condition are elephantiasis and barely detectable ankle, foot, and toe swelling. The edema is painless, "white," and difficult to compress.

Conventional lymphography by Kinmonth (12) provided a solid morphological basis for understanding different disease modalities. It depicts large lymphatic collectors draining the interstitial fluid toward the lymph nodes and into the large abdominal and thoracic ducts. A major limiting factor of the technique has been its traumatic nature requiring incision and cannulation of vessels at the foot dorsum. At present, its use is limited to special diagnostic problems outlined later on.

More recently, two techniques have been developed for staining lymphatic microvessels previously not accessible to human studies in vivo: fluorescence microlymphography with FITC-dextran 150,000 (2, 10) and indirect lymphography with water-soluble contrast media (13, 16). Initial lymphatics or lymphatic capillaries are colored from a macromolecular fluorescent dye deposit in the subepidermal layer (see Chapter 1.4), and the larger precollectors and collectors depicted after subepidermal infusion of the contrast media. In principle, the combination of the three methods mentioned permits visualization of all essential lymphatic vessels.

Because the two techniques depicting lymphatic microvessels are much less traumatic than conventional lymphography, they open a way to confirming different disease modalities and to clarifying complex forms of edema with mixed origin. However, the two procedures have not yet been used in all the important diseases causing edema. For example, no data are currently available for diabetes, myxedema, and cardiac and nephrotic edema. Before establishing the diagnosis case history, relevant clinical findings and laboratory tests should be con-

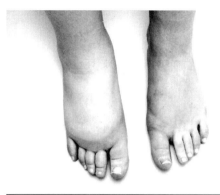
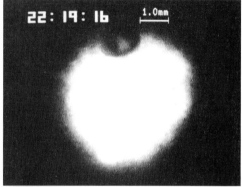
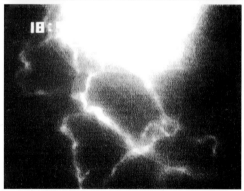

Figure 80. Unilateral congenital and hereditary lymphedema (Nonne-Milroy's disease) in a teenager.
Top: White and painless foot and ankle swelling on the right side. *Middle:* Dye deposit at the right medial ankle: No initial lymphatics are identified. *Bottom:* On the left normal side, several meshes of microlymphatics are colored by FITC-dextran 150,000.

Chapter 2.4

Figure 81. Ectatic form of congenital lymphedema.
Above: Cutaneous reflux far away from the depot (not shown).
Below: The image at larger magnification reveals lymphatic microvessels of increased diameter and irregular caliber. Around the microlymphatics fluorescent spots are stained. They may correspond to filled prelymphatic spaces around blood capillaries (see **Figure 77**).

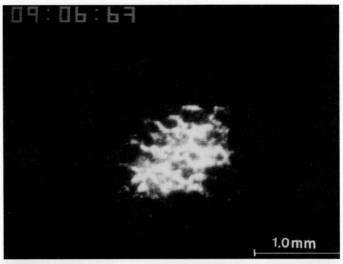

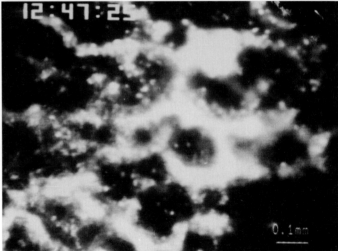

sidered. The results of fluorescence microlymphography or indirect lymphography help to confirm the diagnosis and to classify different subgroups of lymphatic edema. More widespread use of the techniques will probably enhance their diagnostic potential.

Nonne-Milroy's Disease

In Nonne-Milroy's disease, lymphedema is present at birth. Genetic studies suggest that the entity is inherited as an autosomal dominant trait with incomplete penetration; it involves males and females almost equally (3, 6, 12).

To date, 12 patients with hereditary congenital lymphedema have been examined by fluorescence microlymphography (3, 15). Their mean age at the day of investigation was 19.1 years (range 0.25–44 years). Four patients belonged to the same family (3) and two were siblings.

Among these 12 patients, eight showed *aplasia* of microlymphatics in the regions in which the edema was manifest (**Figure 80**). In all cases, several deposits of FITC-dextran

150,000 failed to depict any lymphatic vessels. Only in nonedematous parts of the limb was it possible to color initial lymphatics (3). This finding was particularly striking in a female student who exhibited normal finger end phalanxes but marked congenital lymphedema of the proximal part of her fingers (14). Microvessels were depicted in the skin of the normal end phalanx but not in the proximal edematous parts of the fingers.

In the remaining four patients, the lymphatic capillaries were enlarged (**Figure 81**). Their diameters, determined by the described morphometric technique (see page 56), exceeded 90 μm and were well above the extreme values measured in healthy controls and in patients with sporadic primary lymphedema (**Figure 82**). As in other forms of lymphedema, the area of the depicted network was significantly (p<0.005) enhanced in patients with ectatic microvessels (15).

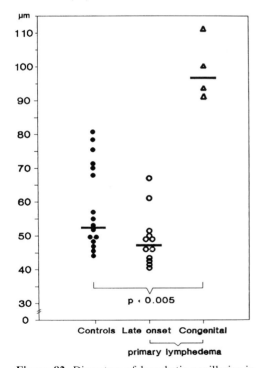

Figure 82. Diameters of lymphatic capillaries in controls, patients with primary lymphedema manifesting after puberty, and patients with ectatic form of congenital lymphedema.

It may be concluded that primary congenital lymphedema is characterized either by aplasia or hyperplasia of microlymphatics. Similar findings were obtained by indirect lymphography (13). The application of the two techniques permits a more accurate diagnosis of Nonne-Milroy's disease. Prognosis and response to therapy could be different in the two disease modalities with aplasia and hyperplasia of skin microlymphatics.

Primary Lymphedema with Manifestation after Puberty

Primary lymphedema manifesting in teenagers and young adults is much more common than Milroy's disease (5, 6). It usually involves the lower extremities of females (male to female ratio 1:5). In about half of the patients, the disease is bilateral. The condition develops sporadically. Only occasionally does the family history reveal a hereditary disease.

Conventional lymphography shows aplastic or hypoplastic large collectors (12). The numeric reduction of vessels and lymph nodes is often confined to the calf and thigh region (distal form). Only rarely do the pelvic vessels participate or are exclusively involved (proximal form).

In contrast to the aplastic or hypoplastic deep collectors, superficial lymphatic capillaries (12) and precollectors (13) are well developed in primary lymphedema with late disease manifestation. The initial skin lymphatics at the medial ankle form an uninterrupted dense and extended network (**Figure 83**). The meshes are tighter at the big toe than at the lower leg (**Figure 84**). In most instances the fluorescence emanating from the microlymphatics is brighter than in normals. Moreover, the filling time of lymphatic capillaries is shortened. Soon after subepidermal injection of FITC-dextran 150,000, the dye rapidly expands into an impressive network.

The dye depicts significantly (p<0.001) larger *areas of the network* than in controls (2, 9, 11, 15). At the medial ankle, mean maximal

Figure 83. Fluorescence microlymphography in a young woman with sporadic primary lymphedema manifesting after puberty.
Above: Depiction of an extended, well-developed network with intact meshes (dye deposit near the bottom). In the right upper part of the image, another network is filled by cutaneous reflux.
Below: Magnification of a network section.

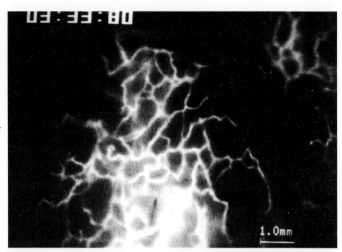

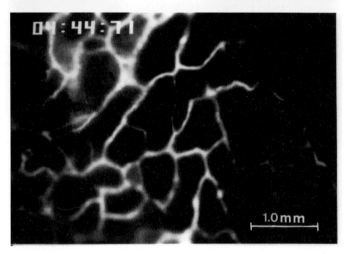

extension of the depicted network measured from the border of the dye depot was 7.8 ± 2.6 mm in normals, but 22.1 ± 13.1 mm in patients (p<0.001). When individual values are considered, there is some overlapping between controls and patients (**Figure 85**). Among 30 patients with primary lymphedema, maximal dye spread did not exceed 12 mm in five patients (9). An extension superior to 12 mm strongly supports the diagnosis of lymphedema, whereas normal findings do not exclude its presence. In seven patients with unilateral lymphedema, fluorescence microlymphography of the opposite unaffected leg was normal in five and pathologic in two instances.

Increased propagation of FITC-dextran 150,000 was also visualized at the big toe in ten patients with primary lymphedema (2, 10). The dye stained almost the entire dorsum of the big toe after placing a deposit of 0.01 ml FITC-dextran 150,000 at the nailfold. In controls, only the lateral part of the toe network was colored.

The increased dye expansion into the superficial network probably results from an impeded drainage of interstitial fluid from the skin into the deeper main collectors. Precollectors are stained by indirect lymphography. They often exhibit valvular insufficiency allowing retrograde flow toward the skin (13).

The phenomenon of *cutaneous backflow*

Lymphedema

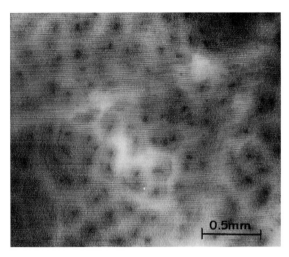

Figure 84. Lymphatic capillary network of a patient with primary lymphedema at the big toe (injection proximal to the nailfold). The meshes are tighter than at the medial ankle. The lymphatic pathways surround one to several blood capillaries (dark points).

may also be demonstrated by fluorescence microlymphography (see **Figures 81** and **83**). In some patients, the fluorescent dye reappears at the surface in islets composed of depicted meshes away from the main network which is in direct connection with the original deposit. It even occurs that a precollector is visualized draining fluorescent material not into deeper channels but into remote superficial areas (11). The presence of cutaneous backflow is an excellent additional diagnostic sign for the diagnosis of lymphedema. To date, the phenomenon has not been reported in normals. On the other hand, it is only observed in a minority of patients with primary lymphedema (9).

The *diameter* of lymphatic capillaries is normal in patients with disease manifestation after puberty (9, 15). Individual and median values are shown in **Figure 82** (15). A clear separation from the values of Milroy's patients with ectatic microlymphatics is apparent. Aplasia or hyperplasia are characteristic for the congenital form, normal caliber of microvessels for sporadic lymphedema manifesting after puberty.

Lymphatic capillary permeability measured by video densitometry (see page 56) is not increased in primary lymphedema (7, 8). As in normals, FITC-dextran 40,000 leaks out of the microvessels, while the larger molecule only occasionally leaves the intravascular compartment. With the molecular size of 150,000, the steep descending curves of the densitometer tracings remain located over the lymphatic capillary wall for 30–60 minutes (8). Microvessels far away from the dye depot were selected for measurement. Differentiation between dye reaching the measuring site from the deposit and through the capillary wall was not a problem like in normals (see page 58).

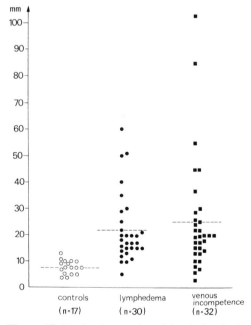

Figure 85. Maximal extension of the depicted microvascular network in one of the four directions at the medial ankle in healthy controls, patients with primary lymphedema manifesting after puberty, and chronic venous incompetence.

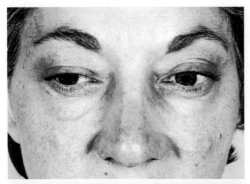
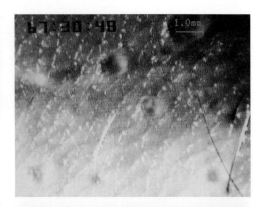
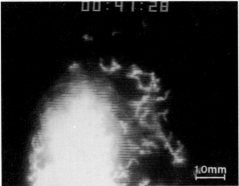
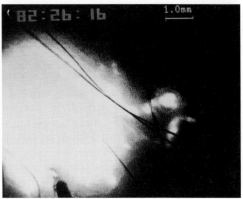

Figure 86.
Above: Patient with lymphedema of the face after recurrent erysipelatas.
Below: Fluorescence microlymphography demonstrates pathologic microlymphatics. The network is fragmented. Some capillaries are not in direct contact with the dye depot but are filled by cutaneous reflux.

Figure 87.
Above: Thigh skin near the groin in a patient with lymphatic hypoplasia of pelvic truncs and lymph nodes. Ruptured blisters evacuate lymphatic fluid.
Below: One saccular enlargement with a diameter of about 0.6 mm is depicted from the depot of FITC-dextran 150,000. It probably corresponds to an unruptured blister.

In contrast to primary lymphedema, damaged microlymphatics in chronic venous incompetence exhibit increased permeability to FITC-dextran 150,000 (see page 103). It is not yet known whether lymphatic microangiopathy after streptococci infection is associated with enhanced leakage.

Pathologic morphology of initial lymphatics was observed in five patients with primary lymphedema complicated by recurrent *erysipelata*. The network may become interrupted by obliterations (**Figure 86**). The morphologic pattern is similar to the one observed in severe chronic venous insufficiency (see page 102).

Probably worsening or first manifestation of the condition after streptococci infection results from secondary damage to the previously normal microlymphatics. Lymphatic microangiopathy becomes an additional factor contributing to edema formation in the presence of hypoplastic large trunks.

In some patients, small blisters develop in the edematous skin (**Figure 87a**). They are filled with lymphatic fluid and may be the origin of lymph fistulae. If FITC-dextran is injected near the blisters, it possibly depicts saccular enlargements of microlymphatics (**Figure 87b**).

Secondary Lymphedema

Secondary lymphedema is caused by the traumatic interruption of lymph collectors, irradiation, or tumor invasion of lymph nodes. Postmastectomy arm lymphedema is a well-known example. In many instances, a time interval is interposed between the underlying trauma or X-ray treatment and the manifestation of disease. In this condition, the lymphatic vessels distal to the site of obstruction are essentially normal. Lymphedema propagates from proximal to distal parts of a given limb. Prestenotic intralymphatic pressure is elevated and induces progressive valvular insufficiency.

Fluorescence microlymphography was performed on the palmar aspect of the lower arm in ten patients with unilateral *postmastectomy lymphedema*. As in patients with primary lymphedema and onset of symptoms after puberty, the dye depicted a larger network on the edematous than on the healthy contralateral side (1). Mean maximal distance between depot edge and most distant meshes filled by FITC-dextran 150,000 was 3.9 ± 2.6 mm on the healthy arm and 70.9 ± 81.3 mm on the arm with secondary lymphedema ($p<0.002$). In one patient with recurrent erysipelata, several subepidermal dye injections failed to visualize any lymphatic microvessel, suggesting destruction of the capillary network by infection. These findings do not permit diagnostic differentiation from primary lymphedema with or without complicating streptococci infections.

As has been described (see page 102) localized secondary lymphedema from CVI is characterized by microangiopathy of blood and lymphatic capillaries. Moreover, microvessel permeability is enhanced in this condition.

General Concept

Fluorescence microlymphography with FITC-dextran 150,000 or tagged human albumin contributes to the establishment of the diagnosis of lymphedema and to the classification of different forms of the disease. **Table 19** summarizes the main findings in different modalities. Differential diagnosis between three important forms of lymphedema can be established:

Table 19. Criteria for differential diagnosis of different forms of lymphedema by fluorescence microlymphography.

	Maximal extension of depicted network	Capillary diameter	Micro-angiopathy	Lymphatic permeability
controls	<12 mm	<90 µm	—	normal
sporadic	>12 mm	<90 µm	—	normal
congenital				
aplastic	—	—	—	—
ectatic	>12 mm	>90 µm	—	?
secondary	>12 mm	<90 µm	—	?
complicating chronic venous incompetence	>12 mm	<90 µm	present	increased
any form complicated by erysipelata	>12 mm	<90 µm	present	?

— sporadic primary lymphedema manifesting in teenagers or young adults,
— aplastic and ectatic form of congenital lymphedema (Milroy's disease),
— local lymphedema secondary to chronic venous incompetence.

However, the technique does not allow differentiation of primary and secondary lymphedema. If there is any suspicion that edema could be the result of neoplastic disease, other diagnostic techniques should be used. Computer tomography or magnetic resonance are able to demonstrate intraabdominal lymphomata causing lymphedema. In the rare cases in which these two noninvasive imaging techniques do not yield conclusive results, conventional lymphography with contrast media should still be used. The decision that primary hypoplasia or aplasia of pelvic vessels and nodes or malignant disease is causing leg swelling is still based on the X-ray procedure. Again, case history and clinical and laboratory findings are important. Elevated blood sedimentation rate in the absence of erysipelata may give rise to suspicion of secondary lymphedema.

References 2.4

1) Baer-Suryadinata, Ch., Clodius, L., Isenring, G., Bollinger, A.: Lymph capillaries in postmastectomy lymphedema. In Bollinger, A., Partsch, H., Wolfe, J. H. N. (eds.), *The initial lymphatics, new methods and findings.* Thieme, Stuttgart, NY, 158–181, 1985.
2) Bollinger, A., Jäger, K., Sgier, F., Seglias, J.: Fluorescence microlymphography. *Circulation* 64, 1195–1200, 1981.
3) Bollinger, A., Isenring, G., Franzeck, U. K., Brunner, U.: Aplasia of superficial lymphatic capillaries in hereditary and connatal lymphedema (Milroy's disease). *Lymphology* 16, 27–30, 1983.
4) Bollinger, A., Partsch, H., Wolfe, J. H. N. (eds.): *The initial lymphatics, new methods and findings.* Thieme, Stuttgart, NY, 1985.
5) Brunner, U.: Klinische Diagnostik des primären Lymphödems der Beine: Erfahrungen an 442 Fällen. *Swiss Med.* 3, 59–66, 1981.
6) Földi, M., Casley-Smith, J. R.: *Lymphangiology.* Schattauer, Stuttgart, 1983.
7) Huber, H., Franzeck, U. K., Bollinger, A.: Permeability of superficial lymphatic capillaries in human skin to FITC-labelled dextrans 40,000 and 150,000. *Int. J. Microcirc.: Clin. Exp.* 3, 59–69, 1984.
8) Huber, M., Hess, U., Bollinger, A.: Measurement of the permeability of cutaneous lymph capillaries in healthy subjects and patients with primary lymphedema. In Bollinger, A., Partsch, H., Wolfe, J. H. N. (eds.), *Initial lymphatics, new methods and findings.* Thieme, Stuttgart, NY, 110-116, 1985.
9) Isenring, G., Franzeck, U. K., Bollinger, A.: Fluoreszenz-Mikrolymphographie am medialen Malleolus bei Gesunden und Patienten mit primärem Lymphödem. *Schweiz. med. Wschr.* 112, 225–231, 1982.
10) Jäger, K., Sgier, F., Seglias, J., Bollinger, A.: Fluorescence microlymphography. *Biblthca. anat.* 20, 712–715, 1981.
11) Jäger, K., Isenring, G., Bollinger, A.: Fluorescence microlymphography in patients with lymphedema and chronic venous incompetence. *Inter. Angio.* 2, 129–136, 1983.
12) Kinmonth, J. B.: *The lymphatics, surgery, lymphography and diseases of the chyle and lymph systems.* E. Arnold, London, 1982
13) Partsch, H., Wenzel-Hora, B. I., Urbanek, A.: Differential diagnosis of lymphedema after indirect lymphography with Iotasul. *Lymphology* 16, 12–18, 1983.
14) Partsch, H., Bollinger, A.: Regionale Hypoplasie dermaler Lymphgefässe—eine neue Variante des kongenitalen Lymphödems. *Wien. klin. Wochenschr.* 98, 704–708, 1986.
15) Pfister, G., Saesseli, B., Hoffmann, U., Geiger, M., Bollinger, A.: Diameters of lymphatic capillaries in patients with different forms of primary lymphedema. *Lymphology* (in print).
16) Wenzel-Hora, B. I., Kalbas, B., Siefert, H. M., Arndt, J. O., Schlösser, H. W., Huth, F.: Iotasul, a water-soluble (non-oily) contrast medium for direct and indirect lymphography. Radiological and morphological investigations in dogs. *Lymphol.* 14, 101–112, 1981.

2.5 Vasospastic Diseases

Primary Raynaud's Phenomenon

Primary Raynaud's phenomenon is characterized by attacks of white fingers provoked by cold exposure or emotional stress. The attacks last for minutes up to one hour and do not lead to trophical changes at the finger tips. Discoloration of fingers is usually bilateral, but does not involve all the digits at the same time. Thumbs are not affected. The male to female ratio is about 1:5. In most patients, symptoms initiate after puberty and tend to regress after menopause. A positive family history is common. Many patients also suffer from migraine, some patients from Prinzmetal's angina pectoris. No underlying disease can be diagnosed. There is no evidence for occlusions of hand or finger arteries. Results of hemorheological (20) and immunological (38) tests are normal.

It is interesting to note that young women exhibit lower mean finger flow than young men and postmenopause women (2). Therefore, a tendency to acral vasospasms is already present in healthy females. Primary Raynaud's phenomenon may be considered as an exaggerated form of normal tendency to vasoconstriction during cold exposure.

Capillaroscopic Findings

Nailfold capillaries are of normal shape and number. Their diameter is normal or slightly enlarged (20, 24, 31). In a Dutch study (20), mean loop diameter at the arterial limb was 16.9 ± 3.7 µm, at the apex 21.6 ± 5.4 µm, and at the venous limb 18.5 ± 4.2 µm. The corresponding mean normal values were 12.9 ± 1.0 µm, 16.9 ± 2.1 µm, and 15.2 ± 1.8 µm, respectively (significant differences at the $p<0.001$ level). However, the increase of capillary diameter is not sufficiently marked to support the diagnosis in single patients.

Blood Cell Velocity

In contrast to acrocyanosis, spontaneous flow pattern in nailfold capillaries is normal. How-

Table 20. Local cooling test: mean capillary flow velocity ($\bar{v}\pm$SD) and flow stop reaction in healthy controls, patients with primary Raynaud's phenomenon (RP), and patients with Raynaud's phenomenon associated with mixed connective tissue disease (MCTD) or scleroderma (Mahler et al., 25).

Clinical diagnosis (mean age)	n female	n male	$\bar{v}$ before cooling (mm/sec)	$\bar{v}$ after cooling (mm/sec)	stop prevalence (%)	stop duration (sec)
Controls (38.9 years)	39	27	0.66±0.10	0.15±0.03+	9/66 (14)	3.4
Primary RP (30.1 years)	7	0	0.27±0.02*	0.01±0.01*+	6/7 (86)*	37.6±11.5*
MCTD (37.3 years)	11	1	0.38±0.17	0.02±0.01*+	11/12 (92)*	59.3±19.7*
Scleroderma (49.5 years)	6	9	0.17±0.10*	0.02±0.01*+	13/15 (87)*	79.5±29.6*

* significantly different from controls ($p<0.01$),
+ significantly different from before cooling ($p<0.01$).

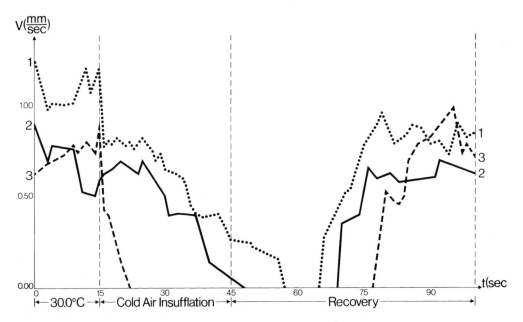

Figure 88. Blood cell velocity (V) in three nailfold capillary loops of a patient with primary Raynaud's phenomenon before, during, and after cold exposure. Flow stop duration varies among the microvessels examined.

ever, blood cell velocity is significantly reduced. Mean blood cell velocity at ambient temperature was 0.66 ± 0.22 mm/s in normals and 0.19 ± 0.19 mm/s in patients with primary Raynaud's phenomenon (p<0.001, 20). In another study (26) the corresponding values were 0.66 ± 0.10 mm/s and 0.21 ± 0.02 mm/s, respectively (**Table 20**).

More drastic changes are observed during and after *cold provocation*. In normals blowing of ice-cooled air at a finger end phalanx for a minute rarely triggers a complete flow stop (3, 24, 25, 27, 28, 32), and if there is a stop, it lasts only a few seconds (25). On the other hand, complete flow stop occurs as a rule in patients with primary Raynaud's phenomenon (25, 32; **Figure 88**). Flow-stop duration is easily determined and used for further characterization of enhanced response to the local cold stress test (26). Mean flow stop was 37.6 ± 11.5 s in primary Raynaud's phenomenon, 79.3 ± 29.6 s in patients with progressive systemic sclerosis, and only 3.4 s in healthy controls (26). A complete flow stop was induced in 9 out of 66 normals, in 6 out of 7 patients with primary Raynaud's phenomenon, and in 11 out of 12 patients with systemic sclerosis. The findings are presented in **Table 20**.

During spontaneous or induced vasospastic attacks, the capillary loops usually remain filled by erythrocytes. Exceptionally, the loops empty and refill at the time of flow restoration (**Figure 89**). It is probable that the bluish discoloration of fingers as a clinical symptom corresponds to red-cell stasis in skin capillaries and the white fingers to emptying of microvessels.

Transcapillary diffusion of NaF is within normal limits. No interstitial areas outside of the pericapillary halo are stained by the dye. Inhomogeneous filling of different capillary groups is found in about one-half of the patients (15).

It may be summarized that borderline enlargement of nailfold capillary loops and pathologic response to cold provocation do not yield specific diagnostic clues (26, 32). The rheologic behavior of blood is normal (20). These findings have to be interpreted together with clini-

Vasospastic Diseases

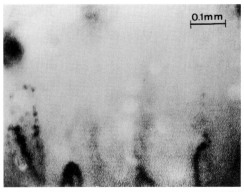

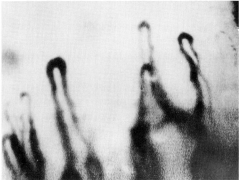

Figure 89.
Above: Partially empty nailfold capillary loops during cold-induced Raynaud's attack.
Below: The same observation field with filled loops after the end of the attack.

cal features and immunological tests. Differential diagnosis with secondary Raynaud's phenomenon is described in the chapter dedicated to connective tissue disease (see page 141).

The absence of microangiopathy favors the diagnosis of primary disease. Indeed, later development of systemic sclerosis is uncommon with normal capillaroscopy (31). Although the enhanced response to cold provocation is not useful for the diagnosis of the condition, it is a good parameter for evaluation of therapy.

Acrocyanosis

Bluish discoloration of fingers and toes which disappears during elevation above heart level is the main symptom of the disease. Acrocyanosis is less common than primary Raynaud's phenomenon, and is usually encountered in young women as well.

Capillaroscopy

The diameter of nailfold capillaries is significantly increased in patients with acrocyanosis (9, 11, 20, 32, 43). However, giant capillaries do not abound as in systemic sclerosis. The enlargement of the loops concerns most of the capillaries visualized (**Figure 90**). Although mean capillary density may be slightly reduced (20), avascular fields are observed only in the rare cases of secondary acrocyanosis from collagen vascular disease or cryoglobulinemia.

Mean capillary diameters and standard deviations were 30.0 ± 8.5 µm at the arterial limb and 34.6 ± 4.2 µm at the venous limb in one study (20), and 18.2 ± 7.3 µm and 21.0 ± 7.9 µm, respectively, in a second study (32). The enlargement of the capillaries in patients with acrocyanosis is more pronounced than in patients with primary Raynaud's phenomenon. The differences between healthy controls and patients are highly significant ($p<0.001$). Moreover, in the study of Jacobs et al. (20), the differences were also significant between primary Raynaud's phenomenon and acrocyanosis ($p<0.001$).

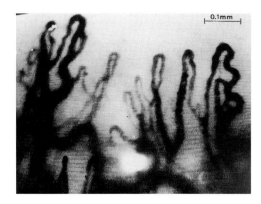

Figure 90. Enlargement of most nailfold capillaries in a female patient with acrocyanosis.

Blood Cell Velocity

The spontaneous speed of blood cells is decreased in acrocyanosis (19, 31). Whereas in healthy controls mean velocity in nailfold capillaries was 0.66 ± 0.22 mm/s, it reached only 0.08 ± 0.05 mm/s in patients (20). This difference is highly significant (p<0.001).

In addition to low flow velocity, nailfold capillaries often exhibit an abnormal *flow pattern* (3, 24, 32). Whereas in healthy volunteers blood cell velocity fluctuates synchronously in adjacent nailfold capillaries, in acrocyanosis the flow pattern in neighboring loops may differ; for example, flow in one capillary is intermittent but low and continuous in an adjacent one. Simultaneously, blood cell speed may accelerate in one given loop and decelerate in the next one (**Figure 91**). Even flow reversal occurs (**Figure 92**). This flow pattern has been called discordant (3, 24, 32).

Response of blood cell speed to a standardized cold provocation test is enhanced (20, 32). Unlike the situation in primary Raynaud's disease, however, there is usually not a uniform decrease of velocity and a flow stop in adjacent nailfold capillaries, but a discordant pattern even during the cold stimulus (3). A typical example is shown in **Figure 92**.

The finding of a delayed and asynchronous arrival of NaF in different nailfold capillaries fits well to the concept of discordant flow pattern. Mean circulation time between arm veins and nailfold capillaries is significantly (p<0.001) prolonged in acrocyanosis (59.3 ± 18.6 s, controls 27.6 ± 6.1 s; 15). In three of six patients it took more than 60 s after first dye appearance until all loops were filled by the dye. Inhomogeneous microvascular flow distribution may be diagnosed, probably as a result of pathologic vasospasms in the precapillary vessels. In addition to a generalized tendency to acral vasospasms (prolonged appearance times of NaF), the spastic changes must be more pronounced in some arterioles than in others inducing discordant flow pattern and inhomogeneous flow distribution.

Capillaroscopic findings are an important element for diagnosing acrocyanosis, a still poorly understood condition. Widespread increase of capillary diameter combined with discordant flow pattern in adjacent loops contributes to establish the diagnosis. When the capillaroscopic image is atypical, secondary disease should be suspected. A thorough clinical investigation, including immunological tests, is then indicated.

Ischemia from Occlusion of Hand and Finger Arteries

There are patients with hand and with finger artery occlusions without evidence of collagen vascular disease. Most of them suffer from arteriosclerosis, endangiitis obliterans, or embolic disease (e.g., thoracic outlet syndrome, hypothenar hammer syndrome). The condition has also be called *asphyxia digitorum* (20). In these patients, symptoms are often limited to some fingers. Raynaud's phenomenon is atypical. The Allen test is positive, and arteriography documents the occlusive lesions.

In patients with arterial occlusive disease and no signs of collagenosis, capillaroscopy is mostly normal. Nailfold loops are regularly shaped and not enlarged (15, 20). However, minor morphologic changes have been described in Buerger's disease (39). Inflow of NaF is not delayed or inhomogeneous (15). Blood cell velocity is decreased at rest without exaggerated response to cold stimuli (3). There is no marked cold hypersensitivity and no increased tone of precapillary vessels as in primary Raynaud's phenomenon, acrocyanosis, and secondary Raynaud's phenomenon resulting from collagen vascular disease (see page 115). It must be realized that a possible decrease in blood cell velocity also depends on time factors. There are no studies yet comparing acute and chronic arterial occlusive disease.

In a unique case with delayed thrombosis in the hand arteries after a 220 V electric shock, the capillary blood cell velocity (CBV) could be measured in the finger nailfold capillaries (5). On the same hand the patient had one finger with a normal blood pressure (120 mmHg), an-

Vasospastic Diseases

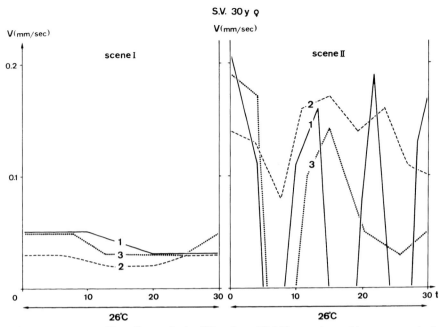

Figure 91. Spontaneous capillary flow velocity (V) at the nailfold in a patient with acrocyanosis. In scene I, low flow velocity is observed in three adjacent loops; in scene II, discordant flow velocity. Capillary 1 exhibits intermittent flow, adjacent capillary 2, continuous flow.

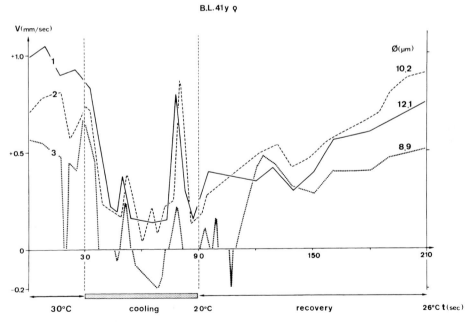

Figure 92. Capillary flow velocity (V) in a patient with acrocyanosis before, during, and after exposure of the nailfold to ice-cooled air. Discordant flow pattern in the adjacent loops is obvious. In the capillary with lowest diameter (Ø), reversal of flow direction is recorded on three occasions.

Figure 93. Finger blood pressure (FBP), postocclusive reactive hyperemia in percent of resting CBV (PRH%), time to peak CBV (tpCBV), and finger temperature before (day 0), during (day 2), and after (day 5) treatment of digital arterial thromboses with streptokinase. ☐: left 4th finger; ■: right 4th finger; ●: right 2nd finger; ○: right 5th finger (reprinted by permission from 5).

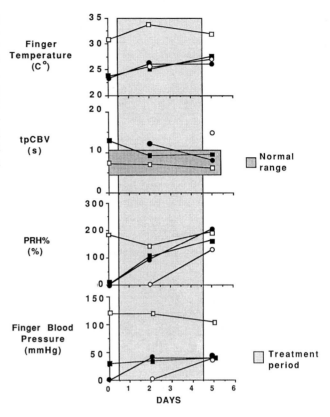

other finger with 30 mmHg, and a third one with 0 mmHg. The skin temperature and CBV during rest and after a 1-minute arterial occlusion was investigated in all three fingers. It was shown that in the fingers with very low pressures, the nutritional capillaries were markedly dilated and slight edema could be seen. During an observation time of half an hour, no blood flow was seen in the capillaries of the fingers with zero and 30 mmHg. These fingers also showed distal prenecrotic changes.

The patient was treated with streptokinase and CBV started on the fifth day of infusion with concomitant improvement of rest pain and necrosis (**Figure 93**). The skin temperature and postocclusive reactive hyperemia response was also markedly improved in the ischemic fingers. This case report shows that the nutritional skin circulation may be completely abolished for days without any necrosis occurring in the area, and when the capillary blood flow starts the ischemic signs can be improved considerably.

Comments: Capillaroscopy of the finger nailfold has only a minor impact for the diagnosis and management of patients with finger artery occlusions without collagen vascular disease or other immunological disorders. Yet, in some patients it may be very helpful for evaluating the effect of therapy on the nutritional blood flow in the ischemic area of these patients.

2.6 Collagen Vascular Disease and Related Disorders

Raynaud's phenomenon often precedes or accompanies collagen vascular disease. Vasospastic changes of precapillary vessels may be associated with arterial occlusive disease of hand and finger arteries (or exceptionally of large vessels), and with microangiopathy. The latter two alterations are lacking in primary Raynaud's phenomenon. Moreover, the typical involvement of visceral organs is not found in primary disease.

Capillaroscopy was already applied in the early 1920s to study capillary morphology of patients with collagen vascular disease (6, 34). The images were drawn and colored by expert artists, since photography was not yet advanced enough to be used with microscopes (**Figure 94**). Later on, the early findings were confirmed (9–11, 24, 43). It was mainly the merit of Hildegard Maricq and coworkers (19, 29–31) to improve the technique and to establish well-accepted criteria for diagnosing microangiopathy. Still more recently, fluorescence video microscopy has increased the diagnostic potential by depicting pathological configuration of pericapillary halos or abnormal interstitial diffusion, and by quantitating enhanced small molecular permeability (1, 4, 36).

Progressive Systemic Sclerosis and Mixed Connective Tissue Disease

The prototype of a disease causing organic and vasospastic arterial changes and in addition capillaropathy is progressive systemic sclerosis or *scleroderma*. In this disease, the prevalence of vascular alterations is inversely proportional to the size of the blood vessels (35). Hand and

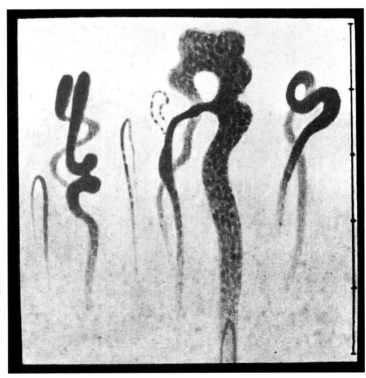

Figure 94. Drawing of nailfold capillaries (1922) by Otfried Müller (33) in a patient with connective tissue disease. The original was painted in color.

finger arteries are often involved (37, 46), but arterioles and capillaries still more frequently.

Microangiopathy has been demonstrated by different histological techniques (13, 21, 35) and in vivo by intravital microscopy with and without fluorescent dyes (1, 2, 4, 6–11, 14, 19, 20, 22–24, 29–31, 33, 34, 38, 43). Cold hypersensitivity was tested measuring red blood cell velocity before, during, and after standardized provocation tests (24–26, 28). Mixed connective tissue disease is commonly associated with microangiopathy that cannot be differentiated from the one observed in scleroderma. Therefore, the two conditions are treated in this chapter.

Evaluation by Conventional Capillaroscopy

The presence of capillaropathy may be suspected by clinical inspection if giant microvessels are obvious. Teleangiectasias are additional clues for clinical diagnosis of microangiopathy. They frequently develop on fingers, toes, face, lip, and mouth mucosa (see **Figure 118,** page 148). Furthermore, spots of white atrophy are not exclusively found in chronic venous insufficiency, but may indicate microvascular involvement in progressive systemic sclerosis or vasculitis of different etiology.

Maricq and coworkers (31) proposed a classification of microvascular changes in patients with systemic sclerosis shown in **Table 21**. It offers a suitable basis for describing the different features of microangiopathy. Typical changes have to be present in at least two finger nailfolds.

Enlargement of nailfold capillaries is the first striking sign of microangiopathy (**Figure 95**). Not all loops are increased in size, however. Microvessels with normal diameter coexist in most instances with definitely enlarged (>20 µm) or giant (>50 µm) loops.

The *loss of capillaries* is the second important condition. Avascular areas may be extensive or localized (**Figure 96**). The surrounding capillaries often lose their normal array. They are oriented toward some of the areas with destroyed microvessels. Ramified capillaries with a "bushy" aspect may be detected. The number

Table 21. Classification of capillary changes in patients with scleroderma and related disorders (modified according to Maricq and coworkers [30]).

Type of nailfold capillaries	I	normal loops
	II	definitely enlarged capillaries with widening of arterial, apical and venous part
	III	giant capillaries (>50 µm)
Loss of nailfold capillaries	A	no obvious avascular area
	B	small avascular areas
	C	moderate loss of capillaries
	D	extensive avascular zone along the edge of the nailfold
Microvascular changes in other skin areas	U	enlarged and ramified capillaries surrounding ulcerations and atrophie blanche spots
	X	capillary teleangiectasias
	Y	diffusely distributed enlarged capillaries

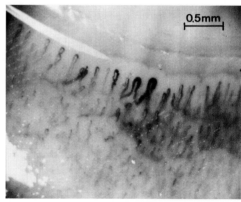

Figure 95. Enlargement of several nailfold capillary loops in a patient with progressive systemic sclerosis. There is no loss of microvessels.

of capillary loops present in 1 mm^2 or in a certain span of the last row may be counted (20). Patients with extreme loss of capillaries tend to have a longer disease duration than those without rarefaction (23). Loss of microvessels has also been documented by histological studies (13, 35).

Collagen Vascular Disease and Related Disorders

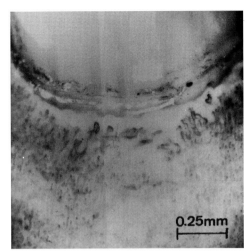

Figure 96. Severe microangiopathy in a patient with progressive systemic sclerosis. Dilatation of loops, irregular arrangement, and avascular areas are apparent.

White atrophy or *atrophie blanche* spots are avascular areas not localized at the nailfold. The avascular field is surrounded by ramified meandering capillaries oriented mostly parallel to the skin surface. The microvessels away from the lesion appear as dots or commas (**Figure 97**).

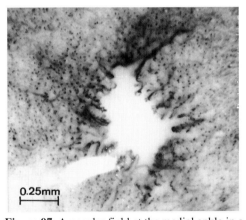

Figure 97. Avascular field at the medial ankle in a patient with progressive systemic sclerosis. The dark spots correspond to loops emerging from below. At the border of the "white atrophy" spot, the capillaries run perpendicular to the skin surface.

Teleangiectasias either contain clusters of enlarged capillaries or are composed of enlarged venules. The latter are less specific for microangiopathy from collagen vascular disease than the widened capillary conglomerates (31). Intravital microscopy reveals teleangiectasias that are not detected by the naked eye.

Pathological examinations show intimal hyperplasia of arterioles and endothelial cell damage (13, 21, 35). The basal laminae are thickened and split up into several layers. Occasionally, obliterated microvessels are encountered.

Changes of the morphologic pattern occur in *follow-up studies* (31). The capillary bed may be reorganized in part. Disappearance and neoformation of loops are both observed. Worsening of microangiopathy is found as a rule, but in exceptional patients microangiopathy disappears (31). This contrasts with normal subjects in whom the pattern of capillary morphology remains fairly constant.

Capillaroscopic findings are of *prognostic relevance*. Follow-up studies suggest that microvascular disease may precede serious involvement of internal organs (14, 31, 38). In fact, it appears to be the best predictor available for the later development of progressive systemic sclerosis. The interval between the diagnosis of microangiopathy and manifestation of other disease symptoms varies between months and many years. The most chronic disease evolution is observed in the CREST variant of scleroderma (16).

"Active" and "slow" scleroderma patterns have been distinguished (31). In the first, reorganization with capillary disappearance and neoformation are detected on repeated examinations. This rapidly changing pattern has been associated with poor prognosis. Disease progressed in five of eight patients during a mean observation period of 3 years. The "slow" pattern consisted of capillary teleangiectasias and/or giant capillaries with no or minimal capillary loss. During 3 years, disease progression was only observed in one out of 11 patients. Large prospective studies are needed to evaluate the prognostic value of these two patterns in more detail.

The *prevalence of microvascular changes* at the nailfold is high in scleroderma. Microangiopathy has been diagnosed in 82% of patients with progressive systemic sclerosis, in 54% of patients with mixed connective tissue disease, and in 2% of patients with lupus erythematosus (30). In another study, 86% of patients exhibited typical capillary changes (23). Markedly increased tortuosity and ramification of capillaries was found in only 6% of scleroderma patients, in 12% of patients with mixed connective tissue disease, and 42% of patients with lupus erythematosus. This finding alone is of questionable diagnostic value.

Since microangiopathy of the "scleroderma-like" pattern occurs in more than 80% of the patients with established disease (23, 30, 38), it is considered to be a valuable *diagnostic tool*. The importance of capillaroscopic findings is supported by the fact that serological tests often fail to reveal significant abnormalities in these patients. The most frequent immunological finding is an increased titer of antinuclear antibodies. In the CREST variant of progressive systemic sclerosis (calcinosis, Raynaud's phenomenon, esophageal dysmotility, sclerodactyly, teleangiectasia), anticentromere antibodies may also be positive. This situation contrasts to lupus erythematosus in which microangiopathy is rare and positive titers of anti-DNA antibodies are common. Serological tests are more useful for diagnosing lupus, capillaroscopic evaluation for diagnosing systemic sclerosis.

According to the criteria advanced by the American Rheumatism Association, progressive systemic sclerosis may be diagnosed in the presence of scleroderma proximal to the digits and/or two of the three so-called minor criteria (sclerodactyly, digital ulceration, bilateral pulmonary fibrosis). Other early clinical signs that may antedate development of the full entity are puffy fingers and digital pitting scars (16). In patients in whom the criteria of the American Rheumatism Association are not fulfilled, microvascular evaluation contributes to establish the diagnosis of *probable scleroderma*. Presence of microangiopathy is an important element. A definitive diagnosis can only be made when the full clinical picture has developed.

Several *limitations* have to be considered. Microangiopathy is not limited to scleroderma and related disorders. It also develops in different conditions like dermatomyositis, Sjögren's syndrome, vibration syndrome, and cryoglobulinemia. Therefore, the presence of microangiopathy requires a thorough clinical examination including appropriate laboratory tests in order to exclude the mentioned diagnostic possibilities.

On the other hand, a simple diagnostic procedure is sufficient when Raynaud's phenomenon without capillary changes is diagnosed. Although the "active pattern" of microangiopathy appears to give some hints for an unfavorable prognosis (31), there is no direct correlation between severity of microangiopathy and organ involvement (23, 33). The time elapsing between the onset of Raynaud's phenomenon and progression to organic disease exceeds 10 years in many patients (14, 38), if it occurs at all. This may be the reason why the follow-up studies performed so far did not document manifestation of generalized disease in all patients with microangiopathy. Only long-term prospective studies have the potential to establish in what percentage of patients with Raynaud's phenomenon and microangiopathy connective tissue disease develops. Microangiopathy appears to have a good predictive value (14, 31, 38), but its full impact is not yet known.

Capillary Blood Cell Velocity at Rest and after Cold Provocation

The velocity of blood cells is decreased at rest in patients with systemic sclerosis (20, 28, 32). At the nailfold, mean velocity was 0.19 ± 0.19 mm/s at rest and 0.032 ± 0.03 mm/s after cold provocation (20). Similar values were determined in another study (26; see **Table 20**).

A standardized cold provocation test using rapidly decompressed CO_2 or ice-cooled air blown on the fingers for one minute demonstrated increased reaction of capillary flow velocity at the nailfold in most of the patients with scleroderma or mixed connective tissue disease (25, 26). The erythrocytes stopped com-

Collagen Vascular Disease and Related Disorders

pletely in 14% of normals, but in 90% of patients. A similar prevalence of cold-induced vasospasms was observed in patients with primary Raynaud's phenomenon. Mean flow-stop duration lasted significantly ($p<0.01$) longer in scleroderma patients than in controls (26). Capillary flow velocity before and after cooling, prevalence of flow stop, and its duration are given in **Table 20**. Cold hypersensitivity is extreme in patients with systemic sclerosis.

Decreased blood cell velocity at rest and during cold stress reflects vasospastic changes. As already pointed out, the different parameters measured during the cold provocation test are pathological in a variety of vasospastic disorders, but they may be used for control of therapy (26). Reduced tendency to vasospastic reactions may be documented by a decrease of mean flow stop time.

Evaluation by Fluorescence Video Microscopy

The use of Na-fluorescein (NaF) (1, 2, 4, 36) or the combination of NaF and indocyanine green (ICG) (7) broadens the criteria available for diagnosis of microangiopathy. The small solute NaF, only partially bound to plasma proteins, diffuses into enlarged pericapillary halos with pathologic shape. It often passes the diffusion barrier at the outer halo border in increased amounts and stains interstitial areas previously invisible. Transcapillary and interstitial diffusion may be quantitated by video densitometry (1, 4). ICG delineates the capillary wall precisely and permits visualization of capillary aneurysms even in the absence of erythrocyte filling (41). Approximate determination of halo diameters becomes possible by combined use of the two tracers (7).

As will be shown, some of the above-mentioned phenomena detected by fluorescent dyes are mainly of scientific interest. However, there are already practical implications. Fluorescence video microscopy enlarges the spectrum of diagnostic information considerably.

— Morphology after Application of NaF

In patients with microangiopathy caused by progressive systemic sclerosis or related disorders, NaF stains pericapillary *halos of abnormal shape*. The halo is mainly enlarged at the apex and assumes a "dwarf hat" aspect (33; **Figures 98** and **108**). The diameter of the pericapillary halo is particularly increased around giant loops.

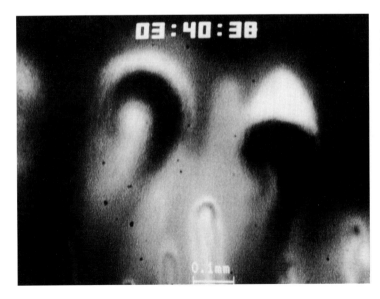

Figure 98. Image of nailfold capillaries obtained by fluorescence video microscopy after injection of NaF in a patient with progressive systemic sclerosis. The loop just above the scale is of normal size and exhibits a well-delineated pericapillary halo. Two giant capillaries are depicted. The enlarged dark column of red blood cells is surrounded by an also enlarged pericapillary halo assuming a "dwarf hat aspect" around the apex of the loop on the right side.

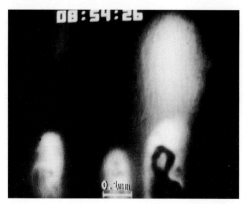

Figure 99. Formation of a large fluorescent "lake" (NaF) outside of the pericapillary halo in a patient with mixed connective tissue disease.

In many instances, the fluorochrome does not respect the *diffusion barrier* at the halo edge and colors interstitial areas (**Figures 99, 100, and 107**). The visual aspect produced by interstitial accumulation of NaF has been described as "street"-, "cloud"- or "lake"-like. The halo border either remains visible or may even be abolished in part or completely (**Figure 100**). Under the latter circumstances, NaF diffuses into the tissue without any additional diffusion barrier. In normals, no dye accumulates in the remote interstitial space. However, microtraumata may damage the barrier function of the outer halo border to some extent. Patients should refrain from manicure several days before examination.

There is an interesting subgroup of patients exhibiting normal or borderline findings at capillaroscopy with white light but definitely pathologic diffusion phenomena (33). **Figure 101** illustrates a typical example and summarizes the three main diagnostic features: normal morphology and dye diffusion (A), normal capillaroscopy without the use of NaF but pathologic transcapillary and interstitial diffusion (B), and giant capillaries with enlarged halo at the apex (C).

Five of the 11 patients belonging to the group with normal morphology and enhanced transcapillary diffusion met the American Rheumatism Association criteria for sys-

Figure 100. Around this giant nailfold capillary, the outer halo border is abolished. NaF diffuses into the interstitial space without barrier (reprinted by permission from 4).
Left: Soon after dye arrival; *right:* 10 minutes after dye arrival.

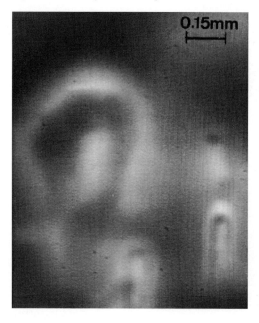
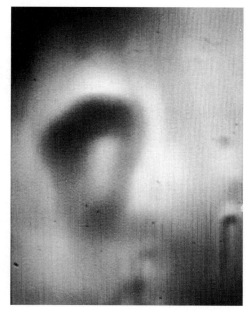

Collagen Vascular Disease and Related Disorders

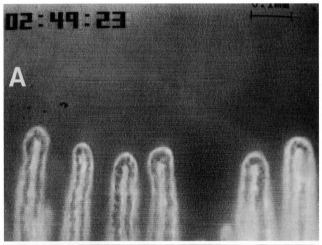
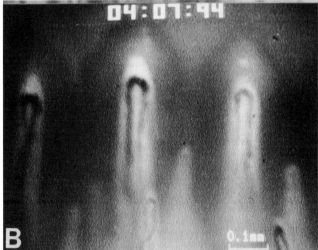
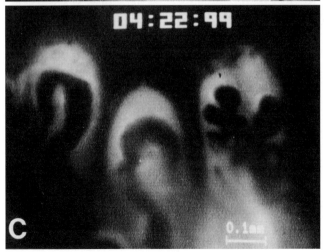

Figure 101. Three main patterns observed by fluorescence video microscopy with NaF.
A) Healthy subject. The dark red cell column is surrounded by a narrow fluorescent compartment containing plasma layer and pericapillary halo.
B) Patient with scleroderma. Normal morphology of capillary loops, but slightly enlarged halos at the apex and increased dye diffusion across the outer border of the halo producing the image of fluorescing "clouds."
C) Patient with scleroderma. Giant loops easily detected by conventional capillaroscopy. Apical capping (enlarged halos) is more pronounced than in image B.

Figure 102. Inhomogeneous inflow of NaF into the nailfold capillary bed and avascular field slowly filled by the dye (young female patient with progressive systemic sclerosis).
Top: 35 s after intracubital dye injection, 6 s after first dye appearance at the nailfold. Large parts of the nailfold are still dark.
Middle: 19 s after first appearance of NaF. In comparison to image above, some more capillaries have been reached by the fluorescent dye. The dark avascular field begins to fluoresce because of dye diffusion from the perfused areas.
Bottom: 1 min 34 s after first appearance of NaF. Diffusion of NaF into the compartment without capillaries renders some venules visible by enhancing the contrast.

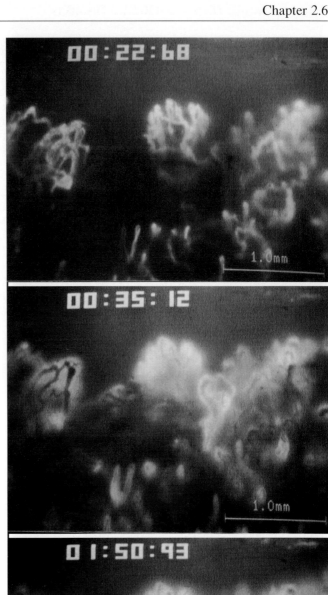
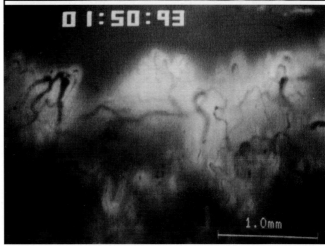

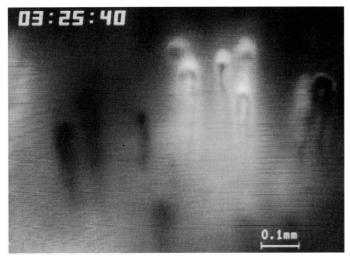

Figure 103. Nailfold capillaries 3 min 25 s after NaF injection and 3 min 3 s after first dye arrival. Among the loops surrounded by the fluorescing material, three dark microvessels containing red blood cells are apparent. They were not filled by NaF during half an hour. Either they are thrombosed or contain long-lasting aggregates of erythrocytes.

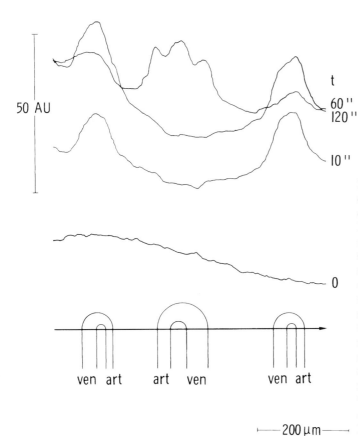

Figure 104. Densitometer curves registered on an axis crossing three adjacent capillary loops shown schematically (arrow). The line indicated by 0's was drawn before arrival of dye (spontaneous fluorescence of the skin). Curves at 10 and 60 s after first NaF appearance show a valley that corresponds to the still empty loop in the middle and two peaks on each side representing capillaries already filled by the dye. At 2 minutes, a third peak appears in the valley ("geyser phenomenon"). It belongs to the capillary filled later. A: arteriolar, B: venular, AU: arbitrary units.

sclerosis (34). In other words, the microangiopathy of these patients would have escaped normal capillaroscopy, but was clearly demonstrated by the fluorescence technique. The use of NaF enhances the diagnostic potential and should be used especially in patients with normal or borderline findings at conventional capillaroscopy (33).

Fluorescence video microscopy is well suited for proving *loss of capillaries*. In fact, the technique stains all the microvessels with flow, even the ones perfused by plasma alone and not by erythrocytes. **Figure 102** gives an example for inhomogeneous inflow of dye and for decreased number of microvessels. In the central part of the image, a black spot without fluorescence is slowly filled up by NaF diffusing into the avascular area of the nailfold from surrounding perfused capillaries. When the interstitium contains enough dye, it fluoresces brightly and contrasts the preserved venules running through the field without capillaries.

Avascular areas probably develop after the thrombotic occlusion of microvessels. As in chronic venous incompetence at the medial ankle (**Figure 74**, page 97), blood-filled capillaries without flow have been detected at the nailfold (**Figure 103**). Some capillaries were not filled by NaF up to half an hour later. This finding corresponds either to red blood cell aggregates trapped in the capillary loops for many minutes or to definitively thrombosed loops.

Microvascular flow distribution evaluated by the time interval between dye filling of the first and last capillaries is pathologic in most patients (15, 33). At the nailfold, the time interval normally lasts no longer than 12 s (see **Table 8**, page 46). A typical example with prolonged time interval is illustrated in **Figure 104**, where fluorescent light intensities were determined on an axis crossing the last row of nailfold capillaries. The last of the three depicted capillaries was only reached by NaF 2 min after first dye appearance.

Like the increased response to a cold provocation test, inhomogeneous distribution of capillary flow is not specific for progressive systemic sclerosis. It has been shown that it also occurs in various other conditions with vasospastic changes and even in severe peripheral ischemia (see **Table 13**, page 71). The inhomogeneous perfusion probably results from intermittent spastic changes of precapillary vessels. An additional explanation is that the rheology of blood is often impaired in patients with secondary Raynaud's phenomenon (20).

Transcapillary and interstitial diffusion of NaF measured by television microscopy and video densitometry is significantly ($p<0.05$–<0.001) increased in patients with progressive systemic sclerosis compared to normal controls (1, 4). In many cases, the abnormal diffusion out of the enlarged microvessels is asymmetrical with respect to the capillary loop. Dye passage may be more enhanced on the arterial or venous limb (**Figure 105**). The steep descending part of the densitometer tracings recorded on an axis crossing the loop at a given distance from the apex (33 µm) corresponds first to the site of the halo border and is displaced later on toward the remote interstitial space. The asymmetrical increase of transcapillary dye diffusion indicates preferential regions of dye leakage along the capillary loop (4) and contrasts to the findings in long-term diabetics (see page 82), where enhanced diffusion through the wall of normally or almost normally looking capillaries is symmetrical.

Diffusion of NaF through the capillary wall is characterized by the values of fluorescent light intensity measured within the pericapillary halo. It is significantly ($p<0.05$–0.001) enhanced in patients with scleroderma (1, 4), signifying that the diffusion barrier formed by the capillary wall is partially abolished. The second diffusion barrier located at the outer halo border is also more permeable for the small solute NaF. Mean fluorescent light intensity is significantly ($p<0.05$–0.01) increased in the remote interstitial space (**Figure 106**). Compared to normal controls, the increase is most significant during the very early phase after dye arrival and is maintained for 20 s.

The mean intraindividual difference of light intensity between the intra- and extrahalo compartment is a direct indicator for the barrier function of the halo border region. A significant

Figure 105. Asymmetrical transcapillary and interstitial diffusion of NaF in a moderately enlarged capillary.
a) Image 1 min 30 s after arrival of NaF at the nailfold. The halo is preserved near the arterial limb of the loop. On the venular limb and at the apex three bright fluorescing spots indicate preferential sites of leakage.
b) Large fluorescing "lake" near the venular side of the loop, still effective barrier for diffusion on the arterial side.
c) Corresponding densitometer curves obtained on a horizontal axis crossing the two capillary limbs 33 μm from the apex at several time intervals from first appearance of dye (reprinted by permission from 4).

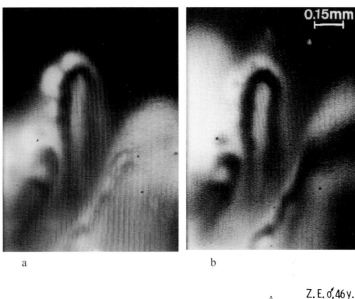

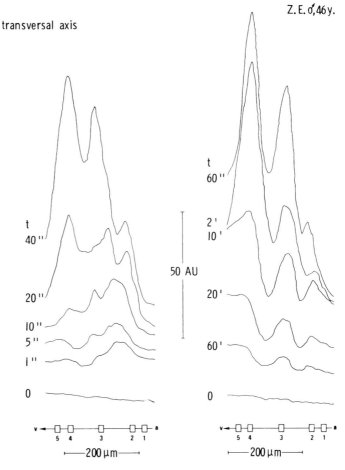

Figure 106. Time/mean fluorescent light intensity diagrams inside (above) and outside (below) the pericapillary halo in 12 healthy controls and 17 patients with scleroderma.
Above: Mean fluorescent light intensities expressed as percentage of the individual maximal intensity near the arterial limb of the loop (site 2). Significant differences are limited to the first 5 s after NaF appearance.
Below: Outside the pericapillary halo (site 1) significant differences persist up to 20 s.

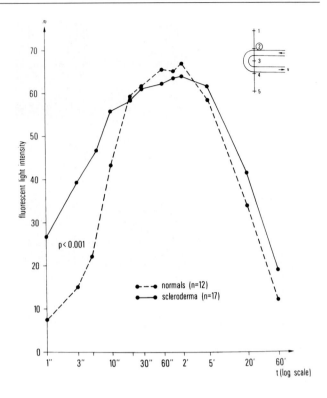

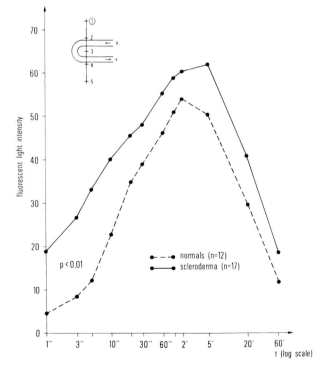

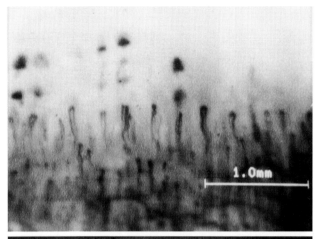
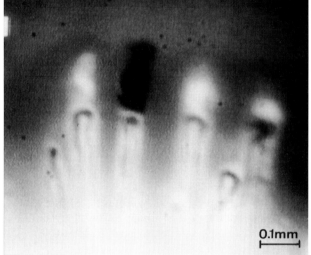
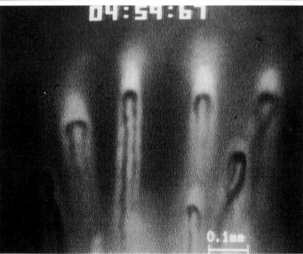

Figure 107. Changing diffusion patterns in a patient who recovered from connective tissue disease that could not be classified precisely. The symptoms were fatigue, general weakness, arthralgias, high sedimentation rate, increased titers of antinuclear and anti-DNA antibodies.
Top: Morphology of nailfold capillary loops at conventional capillaroscopy does not reveal clear signs for microangiopathy.
Middle: However, there is increased diffusion of NaF across the outer halo border. The dark mass at the apex of the third capillary corresponds to microbleeding.
Bottom: One year later, the symptoms had subsided. Titers of anti-DNA antibodies dropped into the normal range. There were no more microbleedings, but still some increased diffusion of the dye into the remote interstitial compartments.

Figure 108. Combination of conventional capillaroscopy (RBC), fluorescence video microscopy with ICG and NaF.
Above: Normal control: Conventional capillaroscopy depicts only the red blood cell column, ICG the real capillary diameter including the plasma layer, NaF halo and red cell column by enhancing the contrast. The latter dye does not delineate the capillary wall in most instances.
Below: Patient with systemic sclerosis. Enlarged capillary loop visualized by both conventional and ICG techniques. Halo enlargement with a typical "dwarf hat" is demonstrated after NaF application.

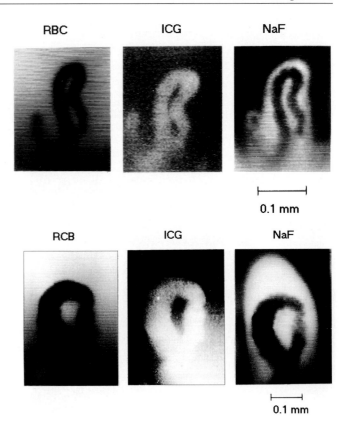

difference between the two values is equivalent with proper function of this second diffusion barrier. In normals, the barrier function at the halo border (significant differences of light intensity) is maintained up to 40 minutes after dye appearance, in patients with progressive systemic sclerosis only up to 1 minute (4).

The hypothesis has been advanced that circulating cytoxic factors or immune complexes damage the endothelial cells and the basal laminae of capillaries inducing enhanced capillary permeability (21). The microedema encircling the loops would then induce activation of myofibroblasts, increased collagen synthesis, and connective tissue fibrosis. According to this theory, microvascular disease is a fundamental event in the pathogenesis of the disease.

To date, no prospective studies have been performed using fluorescence video microscopy. The evolution of diagnostic parameters like halo enlargement or increased transcapillary and interstitial diffusion of NaF is unknown. In first examples, changing diffusion patterns were documented (**Figure 107**).

— **Halo Diameters**

As described in a previous chapter (see **Table 7**, page 45), the dual-tracer technique combining the use of ICG and NaF allows one to assess diameters of full capillary and plasma layer, and to estimate halo size (7).

The mean values determined in 12 patients with progressive systemic sclerosis and related disorders were compared to the data measured in 12 healthy controls (7); they are plotted in **Table 22**. Although the mean halo diameters at the arterial and venous side of the capillary loop were considerably larger in patients than in controls, the values did not differ significantly, probably because of extremely high standard

Collagen Vascular Disease and Related Disorders

Table 22. Mean diameters and standard deviations of capillary (D), red cell column (RBC), plasma layer (PL) and halo (H) at the nailfold in patients with progressive systemic sclerosis (n = 12) and in healthy controls (n = 12) according to Brülisauer and Bollinger (7).

	Arteriolar side			Venular side		
	Patients	Controls	p value	Patients	Controls	p value
D	43.3±21.9	17.7±3.6	<0.001	48.7±27.0	20.4±3.7	<0.001
RBC	32.6±20.6	12.3±2.9	<0.001	36.7±24.6	13.5±3.5	<0.001
PL	10.7± 3.6	5.4±2.4	<0.001	11.9± 4.3	6.9±2.9	<0.005
H	22.5±19.1	8.3±4.5	>0.1	21.6±26.2	8.0±4.1	>0.1

	Apex		
	Patients	Controls	p value
D	55.7±16.3	29.4±4.2	< 0.001
RBC	39.0±15.2	18.5±5.4	< 0.001
PL	16.8± 7.2	10.9±5.8	< 0.03
H	40.3±41.2	9.0±5.8	< 0.01

The values are given in μm.

deviations. At the apex, however, where the visual impression of "dwarf hat" formation is created, mean halo diameter reached 40.3 ± 41.2 μm and was significantly (p<0.01) larger than the normal mean value of 9.0 ± 5.8 μm. A typical example is shown in **Figure 108**. The same capillary was depicted by conventional capillaroscopy and fluorescence video microscopy with NaF and ICG.

In the patients with scleroderma or related disorders, the other three microvascular dimensions (diameters of capillary, red blood cell column, and plasma layer) were significantly augmented at the three sites of measurement (p<0.03–p<0.001). These values were determined at standardized skin temperature (7). By this procedure, possible differences of flow velocity in controls and patients influencing plasma skimming were minimized.

— **Microaneurysms**

Two different types of capillary aneurysms have been defined (**Figure 109**): aneurysms exhibiting a smaller neck and a larger head were called type I (saccular aneurysms). Type II lesions are characterized by a capillary diameter at any part of the loop that exceeds or equals three times the diameter of the smallest loop segment (41).

Since ICG well depicts the inner surface of the capillary wall, it is best suited to visualizing capillary aneurysms (7, 41). Saccular aneurysms may or may not contain red blood cells. They are only suspected by conventional capillaroscopy when erythrocytes whirl outside the

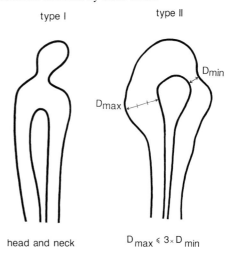

Figure 109. Definition of type I and type II capillary aneurysms. Type I changes are characterized by head and neck. In type II aneurysms, the maximum diameter of the loop equals or exceeds the minimum diameter by three times.

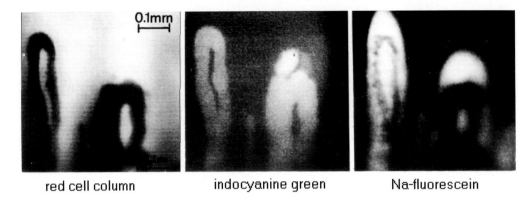

| red cell column | indocyanine green | Na-fluorescein |

Figure 110. Capillary aneurysm type I detected by the ICG technique only. The aneurysm located at the apical part of the enlarged capillary of a patient with scleroderma is not visualized by conventional capillaroscopy since it is not filled by erythrocytes. Fluorescence video microscopy with NaF fails also to stain the aneurysm within a brightly fluorescing halo.

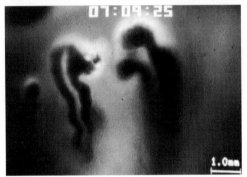
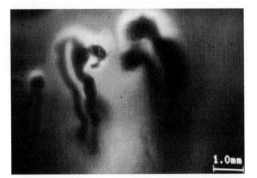
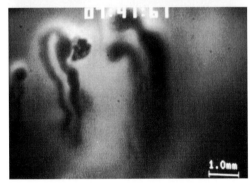

Figure 111. Capillary aneurysm visible with conventional capillaroscopy and the NaF technique. In the three images, NaF enhances the contrast for the moving red blood cells in a nailfold capillary of a patient with progressive systemic sclerosis.
Above: The aneurysm located at the beginning of the venous loop limb is densely filled by erythrocytes.
Above right: The configuration of the red cells in the aneurysm has changed.
Below right: Red cells whirling within the aneurysm provide still another aspect.

main corpuscular stream. Yet diagnosis remains uncertain in most instances. Only after injection of ICG are microaneurysms detected reliably (**Figure 110**). They are mostly located at the apex of the loop and may exhibit a regular or irregular shape. About 50% are filled by plasma alone.

Like conventional capillaroscopy, fluorescence video microscopy with NaF does not allow an accurate diagnosis of microaneurysms. A bright fluorescent spot outside of the dark erythrocyte column may correspond to a preferential site of increased leakage or to a capillary aneurysm. Again, whirling of erythrocytes outside the normal erythrocyte column may indicate presence of a microaneurysm (**Figure 111**).

Although fluorescence video microscopy with ICG appears to be the only technique available to depict capillary aneurysms accurately, some sources of erroneous interpretation have to be considered. The fluorescent light emanating from ICG circulating in the capillary loops is not very intensive, so that the edges of the capillary wall may not be sharply delineated in some instances. This limitation may be overcome in the future by novel techniques of image enhancement and by further improvement of infrared fluorescence video microscopy. Other sources of error include tortuous loops suggesting apical aneurysm formation, occasional superposition of two capillary loops, and the subjective decision whether head and neck are present or not (borderline cases).

The diagnostic relevance of capillary aneurysms is not yet clear. At the nailfold, they occur more frequently in patients with collagen vascular disease and in particular with progressive systemic sclerosis than in healthy controls ($p<0.02$) (41). In normals, the prevalence of type I lesions was 2 out of 12 (17%), and in patients with connective tissue disease 21 out of 38 (55%). Type II aneurysms were diagnosed in 30 patients (79%) and in three controls (25%). This difference of prevalence was also significant ($p<0.001$). A combination of type I and type II aneurysms was found in all 21 patients (55%) exhibiting type I aneurysms. In other words, the two aneurysmatic changes were most often combined. Only in nine patients were type II aneurysms diagnosed without the presence of type I changes. No control subject had a combination of both forms of microaneurysms.

At first sight the detection of capillary aneurysms in healthy controls is surprising. Probably, the ectasias originate from traumata that often occur at the nailfold. The increased prevalence in collagen vascular disease suggests that they are an important feature in microangiopathy of skin. Microaneurysms are well-known elements of retinopathy, particularly in diabetes. No studies have been performed yet to determine the prevalence of skin microaneurysms in this latter disease.

Dermatomyositis

Microangiopathy is common in dermatomyositis. All six patients examined so far in our laboratory exhibited marked to extreme ramification of enlarged nailfold capillaries, loss of loops, and increased transcapillary diffusion of NaF (**Figure 112**). Because dermatomyositis is a relatively rare condition, no prevalence data have been published.

The combination of Raynaud's phenomenon, muscular tenderness and weakness, elevated serum creatine phosphokinase, and positive findings at capillaroscopy is almost pathognomonic for the disease. Per se, microangiopathy cannot be distinguished from the changes observed in progressive systemic sclerosis. Extreme ramification of nailfold capillaries appears to be particularly frequent in this condition (**Figure 112**).

Eosinophilic fasciitis

A normal capillary pattern is found in more than 80% of patients with eosinophilic fasciitis (40). However, there are cases with microvascular involvement resembling the changes observed in progressive systemic sclerosis (17).

Lupus erythematosus

As already mentioned, microangiopathy has a high prevalence in progressive systemic sclerosis and mixed connective tissue disease, but a low prevalence in lupus erythematodes. In the latter disease, microvascular changes at the nailfold were found in only 2% of patients (30).

Because of lacking systematic studies, it is unknown whether fluorescence video microscopy is able to increase the diagnostic potential of conventional capillaroscopy. **Figure 113** gives an example for marked microangiopathy in a young woman with lupus erythematosus. In this case, giant capillaries and a moderate rarefaction of microvessels were evident.

Chapter 2.6

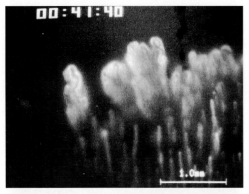

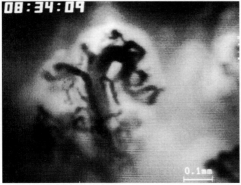

Figure 112. Fluorescence video microscopy with NaF in a patient with dermatomyositis.
Above: Low magnification showing extremely ramified microvessels at the nailfold. Blurring indicates increased transcapillary diffusion.
Below: High magnification with a large capillary resembling a tree.

As a general rule, and at the present state of the art, capillaroscopy contributes to the diagnosis of lupus erythematosus only in exceptional cases. Clinical findings, serological tests, and in particular the presence of DNA antibodies must guide the clinician.

Rheumatoid Arthritis

Occasionally, microangiopathy at the nailfold has been diagnosed in patients with rheumatoid arthritis, especially in its seropositive form. A systematic study (18) including 11 patients with osteoarthritis as group of comparison, 13 patients with seronegative, and 10 patients with seropositive disease revealed no major morphologic changes of microvessels even after application of NaF. Transcapillary diffusion of NaF and pericapillary halo shape were normal. It must be emphasized that the study did not contain patients with vasculitis.

Spontaneous mean blood cell velocity was significantly decreased in the seropositive group of patients ($p<0.02$). It was 0.59 ± 0.20 mm/s in osteoarthritis, 0.35 ± 0.17 mm/s in seronegative and 0.23 ± 0.21 mm/s in seropositive rheumatoid arthritis (18).

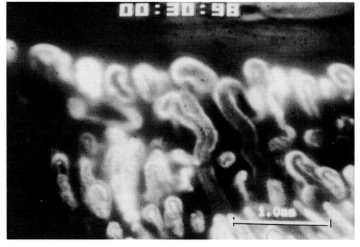

Figure 113. Microangiopathy of a young female patient with lupus erythematosus suffering from severe finger ischemia. Widened and tortuous loops abound at the end-row of the nailfold. The more proximal capillaries are of almost normal size (fluorescence video microscopy 31 s after NaF injection and 11 s after first dye arrival).

Vibration Disease

Working with vibrating tools for long periods of time may induce Raynaud's phenomenon. In patients using chain saws, the number of visible capillaries at the last row of the nailfold was significantly decreased (9.9 ± 2.1 loops/mm) compared to controls (11.7 ± 1.6 loops/mm). Moreover, prevalence of pericapillary hemorrhages was enhanced in these patients (42). In this particular condition, easily recognized by careful case history, vasospastic and organic changes of the microcirculation overlap. Reduced tolerance to cold stress is objectively assessed by the tests described earlier.

Cytostatic Therapy with Bleomycin and Vinblastine

This treatment commonly induces Raynaud's phenomenon (44). Even progression to digital gangrene has been described (12). In 12 young patients (mean age 28.2 years) treated for germ cell carcinoma, fluorescence video microscopy was performed and the findings compared to those obtained in 12 healthy controls (mean age 31.2 years). The patients received a mean total amount of 315.8 ± 61.6 mg (range 180–385 mg) bleomycin, 74.6 ± 42.6 mg (26–200 mg) vinblastine and 567.7 ± 197 mg (360–1080 mg) cis-platin. Three of the 11 men (one woman was also included) developed Raynaud's phenomenon and four a tendency toward cold fingers not present before cytostatic therapy was initiated (45).

In the patients, the diameter of red blood cell column averaged 11.9 ± 1.9 μm on the arterial limb of the nailfold capillaries and 15.8 ± 2.2 μm on the venous limb. The corresponding values in the controls were 10.1 ± 2.0 μm and 13.1 ± 2.7 μm, respectively. Although significant ($p<0.05$) the enlargement of the nailfold loops was not pronounced. In these patients, no capillary loss and no increased prevalence of giant capillaries was noted.

Appearance time of NaF at the nailfold was normal, but the time interval between filling of the first and last capillaries significantly prolonged ($p<0.002$). In the controls, the mean interval was 6.8 ± 3.7 s, in the patients 20.6 ± 12.3 s (45). Unequivocal abnormalities of transcapillary and interstitial diffusion were not observed.

It may be concluded that cytostatic therapy with bleomycin and vinblastine in the dosage described induces vasospastic changes of the precapillary vessels and minor enlargement of capillaries. There was no clear correlation between clinical symptoms (Raynaud's phenomenon, cold hands and fingers) and microangiopathy.

Cryoproteinemia

Circulating cryoproteins cause systemic symptoms such as arthralgias, neuropathy or nephritis, and vascular symptoms including Raynaud's phenomenon, acral necrosis, or purpura. The disease is either idiopathic or part of an underlying disorder (collagen vascular disease, plasmocytoma, malignant lymphoma).

Intravital microscopic observations in cryoproteinemia are scarce. In an own case presenting with Raynaud's phenomenon and purpura (8), abundant microbleedings were evident at the finger dorsum and at the nailfold. After injection of NaF, the dye reached some capillaries early, but large areas were not filled by the dye even 10 minutes later (**Figure 114**). The fluorescent tracer promptly diffused out of the intravascular compartment causing early blurring of the capillary outlines. Electron optic studies disclosed fibrin clots obstructing some microvessels and marked endothelial cell damage in the vessels still patent (8).

At a second study performed 5 weeks later, all the nailfold microvessels of the identical finger were homogeneously filled. No microbleedings were visualized. Transcapillary diffusion seemed still somewhat enhanced. Clinical symptoms had subsided after systemic treatment with corticosteroids.

Table 23. Microvascular diagnostic criteria in Raynaud's phenomenon (RP) and acrocyanosis.

	Normals	Primary RP	RP due to scleroderma	Acrocyanosis
capillary diameter	normal	slightly enlarged	enlarged with giant capillaries	enlarged
rarefaction of capillaries	lacking	lacking	present	lacking
spontaneous flow velocity	normal	normal or slightly decreased	decreased	decreased
flow velocity pattern	concordant	concordant	discordant	discordant
velocity reaction to cold stimulus	normal	flow stop	flow stop	irregular
flow distribution	homogeneous	homogeneous or slightly nonhomogeneous	non-homogeneous	non-homogeneous
halo morphology	normal	normal	"dwarf hat"	normal
transcapillary diffusion	normal	normal	enhanced	normal
interstitial diffusion	normal	normal	"cloud"-like accumulation	normal

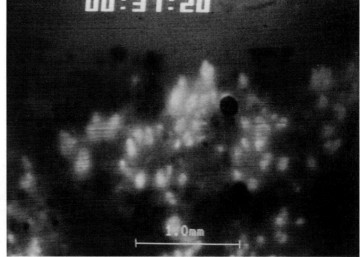

Figure 114. Finger capillaries of a patient with essential cryoproteinemia. The dark parts not reached by NaF correspond to microbleedings or areas with obliterated microvessels (8).

Concluding Remarks

Table 23 summarizes the microvascular diagnostic criteria useful for the clinician confronted with Raynaud's phenomenon or acrocyanosis. Capillaroscopy is a valuable tool for a correct diagnosis, provided that clinical, serological, and immunological findings are considered as well. The absence of microangiopathy strongly supports the presence of primary Raynaud's phenomenon, when patients with hand and finger artery occlusions are excluded by other appropriate means.

If microangiopathy is present, the most likely diagnoses are progressive systemic sclerosis, mixed connective tissue disease and dermatomyositis. The latter condition is characterized by muscular pain, weakness and high levels of creatine phosphokinase. In the rare cases in which microangiopathy develops in systemic lupus erythematodes, anti-DNA antibodies are found. Microangiopathy in combination with stiff puffy fingers, but not fulfilling the criteria of the American Rheumatism Association, is a fairly good predictor for later development of scleroderma. Raynaud's phenomenon from the use of vibrating tools and from therapy with bleomycin or vinblastine is easily recognized without microvascular examination.

Fluorescence video microscopy enhances the diagnostic potential of conventional capillaroscopy by 10–15% (33). About 80% of cases with microangiopathy from scleroderma are identified without application of fluorescent tracers (30).

References 2.5 and 2.6

1) Bollinger, A., Jäger, K.: Trans- and pericapillary diffusion of Na-fluorescein in scleroderma and chronic venous insufficiency. *Biblthca. anat.* 20, 679–683, 1981.
2) Bollinger, A.: Contribution of dynamic microvascular studies to pathophysiology and diagnosis of Raynaud's phenomenon. *Adv. Microcirc.* 12, 82–94, 1985.
3) Bollinger, A.: Function of the precapillary vessels in peripheral vascular disease. *J. Cardiovasc. Pharmacol.* 7 (Suppl. 3), S147–151, 1985.
4) Bollinger, A., Jäger, K., Siegenthaler, W.: Microangiopathy of progressive systemic sclerosis, evaluation by dynamic fluorescence video microscopy. *Arch. Int. Med.* 146, 1541–1545, 1986.
5) Bongard, O., Fagrell, B.: Delayed arterial thrombosis following an apparently trivial low-voltage electric injury. *VASA* 18, 162–166, 1989.
6) Brown, G. E.: The skin capillaries in Raynaud's disease. *Arch. Int. Med.* 35, 56–73, 1925.
7) Brülisauer, M., Bollinger, A.: Measurement of different human microvascular dimensions by combination of video microscopy with Na-fluorescein (NaF) and indocyanine green (ICG) in normals and patients with systemic sclerosis. *Int. J. Microcirc.: Clin. Exp.* (in print).
8) Brüngger, A., Brülisauer, M., Mitsuhashi, Y., Schneider, B. V., Bollinger, A., Schnyder, U. W.: Cryofibrinogenemic purpura. *Arch. Dermatol. Res.* 279, 24–29, 1987.
9) Carpentier, P., Franco, A.: *La capillaroscopie périunguéale.* Deltacom, Paris, 1981.
10) Cervini, C., Grassi, W., Gasparini, M., Cervini, M.: Il microcircolo nella sclerosi sistemica. *Acta Cardiol. Medit.* 3, 87–95, 1985.
11) Davis, E., Landau, J.: *Clinical capillary microscopy.* Thomas, Springfield, 1966.
12) Elomaa, I., Pajunen, M., Virkkunen, P.: Raynaud's phenomenon progressing to gangrene after vincristine and bleomycin therapy. *Acta Med. Scand.* 216, 323–326, 1984.
13) Fiessinger, J. -N., Amilleri, J. -P., Mignot, J., Kazandjian, S., Vayssairat, M., Housset, E.: La microangiopathie sclérodermique–hypothèses physiopathogéniques. *Rev. Méd. Int.* 1, 61–64, 1980.
14) Fitzgerald, O., Hess, E. V., O'Connor, G. T., Spencer-Green, G.: Prospective study of the evolution of Raynaud's phenomenon. *Am. J. Med.* 84, 718–726, 1988.
15) Franzeck, U. K., Isenring, G., Frey, J., Bollinger, A.: Video densitometric pattern recognition of Na-fluorescein diffusion in nail-

fold capillary areas of patients with acrocyanosis, primary vasospastic and secondary Raynaud's phenomenon. *Inter. Angio.* 2, 143–152, 1983.

16) Gerbracht, D. D., Steen, V. D., Ziegler, G. L., Medsger, T. A., Rodnan, G. P.: Evolution of primary Raynaud's phenomenon (Raynaud's disease) to connective tissue desease. *Arthritis Rheum.* 28, 87–92, 1985.

17) Grassi, W., Gasparini, M., Cervini, C.: Nailfold capillary microscopy in eosinophilic fasciitis–report in two cases. *Conn. Tiss. Dis.* 3, 29–33, 1984.

18) Grassi, W., Felder, M., Thüring-Vollenweider, U., Bollinger, A.: Microvascular dynamics at the nailfold in rheumatoid arthritis. *Clin. Exp. Rheumatol.* 7, 47–53, 1989.

19) Harper, F. E., Maricq, H. R., Turner, R. E., Lidman, R. W., Leroy, E. C.: A prospective study of Raynaud's phenomenon and early connective tissue disease–A five-year report. *Am. J. Med.* 72, 883–888, 1982.

20) Jacobs, M. J. H. M., Breslau, P. J., Slaaf, D. W., Reneman, R. S., Lemmens, J. A. J.: Nomenclature of Raynaud's phenomenon–A capillary microscopic and hemorheologic study. *Surgery* 101, 136–145, 1987.

21) Jayson, M. I. V.: Systemic sclerosis–A microvascular disorder ? *J. Roy. Soc. Med.* 76, 635–642, 1983.

22) Kimby, E., Fagrell, B., Björkholm, M., Holm, G., Mellstedt, H., Norberg, R.: Skin capillary abnormalities in patients with Raynaud's phenomenon. *Acta Med. Scand.* 215, 127–134, 1984.

23) Lovy, M., MacCarter, D., Steigerwald, J. C.: Relationship between nailfold capillary abnormalities and organ involvement in systemic sclerosis. *Arthritis Rheum.* 28, 496–501, 1985.

24) Mahler, F., Bollinger, A.: Die Kapillarmikroskopie als Untersuchungsmethode in der klinischen Angiologie. *Dtsch. med. Wschr.* 103, 523–527, 1978.

25) Mahler, F., Saner, H., Annaheim, M., Linder H. R.: Capillaroscopic examination of erythrocyte velocity in patients with Raynaud's syndrome by means of a local cold exposure test. *Prog. appl. Micorcirc.* 11, 47–59, 1986.

26) Mahler, F., Saner, H., Boss, Ch., Annaheim, M.: Local cold exposure test for capillaroscopic examination of patients with Raynaud's syndrome. *Microvasc. Res.* 33, 422–427, 1987.

27) Maricq, H. R., LeRoy, E. C.: Capillary blood flow in scleroderma. *Bibl. anat.* 11, 352–358, 1973.

28) Maricq, H. R., Downey, J. A., LeRoy, E. C.: Standstill of nailfold capillary blood flow during cooling in scleroderma and Raynaud's syndrome. *Blood Vessels* 13, 338–349, 1976.

29) Maricq, H. R., LeRoy, E. C.: Progressive systemic sclerosis–disorders of the microcirculation. *Clin. Rheum. Dis.* 5, 81–101, 1979.

30) Maricq, H. R., LeRoy, E. C., D'Angelo, W. A., Medsger, T. A., Rodnan, G. P., Sharp, G. C., Wolfe, J. F.: Diagnostic potential of in vivo capillary microscopy in scleroderma and related disorders. *Arthritis Rheum.* 23, 183–189, 1980.

31) Maricq, H. R., Harper, F. E., Khan, M. M., Tan, E. M., LeRoy, E. C.: Microvascular abnormalities as possible predictors of disease subsets in Raynaud phenomenon and early connective tissue disease. *Clin. Exp. Rheumat.* 1, 195–205, 1983.

32) Meier, B., Mahler, F., Bollinger, A.: Blutflussgeschwindigkeit in Nagelfalzkapillaren bei Gesunden und Patienten mit vasospastischen und organischen akralen Durchblutungsstörungen. *VASA* 7, 194–198, 1978.

33) Moneta, G., Vollenweider, U., Dubler, B., Bollinger, A.: Diagnostic value of capillaroscopy with and without fluorescent dyes to detect early connective tissue disease. *VASA* 15, 143–149, 1986.

34) Müller, O.: *Die Kapillaren der menschlichen Körperoberfläche in gesunden und kranken Tagen.* Enke, Stuttgart, 1922.

35) Norton, W. L., Nardo, J. M.: Vascular disease in progressive systemic sclerosis (scleroderma). *Ann. Int. Med.* 73, 317–324, 1970.

36) Pilger, E.: Computergestützte In-vivo-Untersuchung der Kapillarpermeabilität. *Wien. Med. Wschr.* Suppl. 94, 2–42, 1985.

37) Porter, J. M., Snider, R. L., Bardana, E. J. et al.: The diagnosis and treatment of Ray-

naud's phenomenon. *Surgery* 77, 11–23, 1975.

38) Priollet, P., Vayssairat, M., Housset, E.: How to classify Raynaud's phenomenon– Long-term follow-up study of 73 cases. *Am. J. Med.* 83, 494–498, 1987.

39) Ranft, J., Heidrich, H.: Vital capillary-microscopic findings in normal subjects, patients with peripheral arterial occlusive disease (Fontaine II to IV) and patients with thrombangiitis obliterans. *VASA* 15, 138–142, 1986.

40) Rozboril, M. B., Maricq, H. R., Rodnan, G. P., Jablonska, S., Bole, G. G.: Capillary microscopy in eosinophilic fasciitis. A comparison with systemic sclerosis. *Arthritis Rheum.* 26, 617–622, 1983.

41) Saesseli, B. F. E.: Fluoreszenz-Video mikroskopie mit Indozyaningrün (ICG): Eine Methode zur intravitalen Detektion von Kapillaraneurysmen. Dissertation, Zürich, 1988.

42) Vayssairat, M., Patri, B., Guilmot, J. L., Housset, E., Dubrisay, J.: La capillaroscopie dans la maladie des vibrations. *Nouv. Presse Med.* 11, 3111–3115, 1982.

43) Vayssairat, M., Priollet, P.: Atlas pratique de capillaroscopie. *Revue de Médecine*, Paris, 1983.

44) Vogelzang, N. J., Bosl, G. J., Johnson, K., Kennedy, B. J.: Raynaud's phenomenon: a common toxicity after combination chemotherapy for testicular cancer. *Ann. Intern. Med.* 95, 288–292, 1981.

45) Weber, D.: Raynaud-Phänomen und videomikroskopische Befunde nach zytostatischer Behandlung von Patienten mit malignen Keimzelltumoren. Dissertation, Zürich 1989.

46) Zweifler, A. J., Trinkaus, P.: Occlusive digital artery disease in patients with Raynaud's phenomenon. *Am. J. Med.* 77, 995–1001, 1984.

2.7 Hematological Disorders

It is well known that hemorheology plays an important role in the circulation of blood through nutritional capillaries (1, 4). It is therefore of great interest to study how the skin capillary circulation is influenced by different diseases affecting the blood hemorheology. In humans, such studies have been performed in polycythemia (2) and leukemia (5).

Polycythemia

Primary Polycythemia

When hematocrit is reduced from very high values, beneficial effects on CBV can be demonstrated, especially in an area with a reduced arterial circulation. The following case report is a good ilustration of this:

A 48-year-old woman was refered to the hospital because of cyanosis and rest pain in digit III and IV of the left hand. On investigation, it was found that the arm blood pressure was equal in the two arms (120/70 mmHg). However, the systolic blood pressure of the left fourth finger was only 70 mmHg in comparison with 110 mmHg in the fourth finger of the right hand. The hemoglobin value was 189 g/l and the hematocrit was 63%. Further investigations revealed that the patient had *polycythemia vera* with platelets of $750 \times 10^3/mm^3$. The patient consequently demonstrated marked polycythemia and had one ischemic and one normal digit to investigate.

rCBV was only 0.01 mm/s in the ischemic hand before hemodilution, but also in the control hand rCBV was extremely low (**Table 24**). After a 1-minute arterial occlusion, it took 16 s (N = 7–11 s) for the blood flow to start in the ischemic finger and 5 s in the normal one (**Figure 115**). This indicates that the blood viscosity

Table 24. CBV in a patient with polycythemia vera and ischemia in the left hand because of arterial obliterations of the digital arteries. In the right hand the arterial circulation was normal.

	Hemodilution			
	Left hand fourth finger before / after		Right hand fourth finger before / after	
Hct (%)	63	39	63	39
rCBV (mm/s)	0.01	0.1	0.02	0.2
PRH start (s)	16	0	4.5	0
tpCBV (s)	43	20	7	5
duration (s)	58	100	10	17
pCBV (mm/s)	0.07	0.28	0.16	0.4
PHR%	600	180	700	100

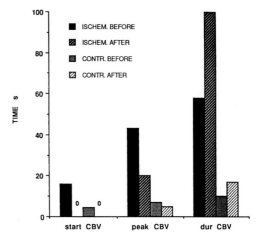

Figure 115. Reaction of CBV during postocclusive reactive hyperemia after a 1-minute arterial occlusion in a patient with polycythemia vera. One of the investigated fingers (ISCHEM) had arterial insufficiency and ischemia, and the other finger (CONTR.) had a normal arterial circulation. Polycythemia seems to affect PRH response in the ischemic finger significantly, while only a minor effect was seen in the nonischemic finger. There is a marked delay in the start of CBV, the time to peak CBV, and also the duration of hyperemia (dur CBV) (see further text on pages 27 and 138–139).

was so elevated, and the resistance to flow so increased, that it took a long time before a high enough intravascular pressure was reached to start the blood flow in the capillaries. The time to peak CBV was also extremely prolonged in the ischemic finger (43 s), but normal in the control fingers (**Figure 115**). After isovolemic hemodilution the hemoglobin and hemotocrit were markedly reduced to 117 g/l and 39%, respectively. rCBV increased 10 times in both fingers, and during PRH a dramatic improvement was seen, especially in the ischemic finger (**Table 24**). Flow started immediately in the ischemic finger after release of the arterial occlusion, and the time to peak CBV decreased from 43 to 20 s. In the nonischemic finger, flow also started immediately and time to peak CBV was still normal (**Figure 115**).

Comments: This case report nicely illustrates that a high hematocrit is detrimental for the microcirculation in ischemic skin areas, and that isovolemic hemodilution can markedly improve the nutritional blood flow in the skin capillaries. On the other hand, the effect on the nutritional blood flow in a nonischemic skin region was very limited, which is in agreement with what has been found in the patients with secondary polycytemia also.

Secondary Polycythemia

The CBV was studied in the finger nailfold capillaries of seven patients with secondary polycythemia due to chronic respiratory disease (2). The patients were investigated immediately before and 2–4 hours after an isovolemic hemodilution during which 500–750 ml of blood was replaced by an equivalent amount of 6% dextran-70 solution (Macrodex®, Pharmacia, Sweden). A control group of seven healthy, age matched subjects with normal hemotocrit values was selected for comparison. The hematocrit was significantly ($p<0.001$) higher in the patients than in the controls. The skin temperature was about 2°C higher (n.s.) in the control subjects. rCBV before hemodilution was equal in the patients and the controls, and there was no significant improvement in skin capillary reactivity.

Comments: In the study presented above, only a moderate isovolemic hemodilution (52%→46%) was performed, which might explain why no significant effect on the CBV values was recorded. The use of dextran-70, which has an equal, or even slightly higher, viscosity than plasma, might also explain the lack of increase in CBV. The optimal effects for microcirculatory flow in a resting tissue have been reported to occur when hematocrit is reduced to values of 30–35% (3).

Leukemia

It is well known in clinical practice that blocking of capillaries causes a decreased perfusion in various organs with damage of tissues, especially the lungs. Through capillaroscopy it is possible to investigate the flow behavior in skin capillaries of patients with very high white blood cell (WBC) counts. It has been shown that the skin microcirculation is impaired in pa-

Table 25. The effect of different kinds of leukemia on CBV ($\bar{x}\pm SD$). Chronic lymphocytic (CLL), and granylocytic (CGL) leukemia.

	CLL n=6	CGL n=11	Controls n=18
WBC count (10^9/l) range	70–542	67–136	4–11
rCBV (mm/s)	0.35 ± 0.10	0.28 ± 0.7*	0.60 ± 0.38
pCBV (mm/s)	0.86 ± 0.23	0.58 ± 0.10***	1.22 ± 0.47
tpCBV (s)	8.2 ± 2	7.7 ± 1	7.4 ± 2.1

p-values compared to controls: * <0.05, *** <0.001

tients with chronic granulocytic leukemia, and this impairment can be improved by cytoreduction (5).

In one study, the influence of different cell types of leukemic cell origin on skin capillary circulation was evaluated in patients with chronic lymphocytic leukemia (CLL), and chronic granulocytic leukemia (CGL). rCBV was found to be significantly lower in patients with CGL, but not significantly so in patients with CLL (**Table 25**). It was shown that in patients with CGL, both resting CBV and peak CBV during postocclusive reactive hyperemia were significantly lower than in healthy controls. The values in the CLL patients did not differ from those in the controls. The clinical symptoms were more marked in patients with low CBV values, especially in the CGL group, and it is therefore suggested that the size of the leucocytes may be a factor of importance for the development of hyperviscosity syndromes and organ malperfusion in leukemic patients.

References 2.7

1) Driessen, G., Heidtman, H., Scheidt, H., Schmid-Schönbein, H.: Effect of hemodilution and hemoconcentration on microcirculation perfusion. *Bibl. Haematol.* 47, 21–30, 1981.
2) Fagrell, B., Östergren, J.: Skin capillary blood cell velocity in patients with arterial obliterative disease and polycythemia–A disturbed reactive hyperemia response. *Clin. Physiol.* 5, 35–43, 1985.
3) Messmer, K., Sunder-Plassmann, L., Klövekorn, W. P., Holper, K.: Circulatory significans of hemodilution. Rheological changes and limitations. *Adv. Microcirc.* 4, 1, 1972
4) Thomas, D. J., Boulay du, G. H., Marshall, J.: Effect of hematocrit on cerebral blood-flow in man. *Lancet* ii, 941–943, 1977.
5) Tooke, J. E., Milligan, D. W.: Capillary flow velocity in leukemia. *Br. Med. J.* 286, 518, 1983.

2.8 Miscellaneous Disorders

Hypertension

Total peripheral resistance (TPR) is increased in most patients with hypertension. However, it is still not known exactly in which vascular bed it is increased. There is evidence that the mechanism responsible for the increase in TPR is mainly localized within the renal and splanchnic vascular bed and not within the muscles (2). However, in a study by Zweifler and Nicholls (22), it was found that the pulse volume in fingers was significantly lower at maximum dilatation in patients with borderline hypertension than in normal subjects. They concluded that the elevation of blood pressure produces structural vascular changes also in the finger vessels. It is therefore of interest to investigate how the microvascular bed of the skin of fingers is influenced by an elevated blood pressure.

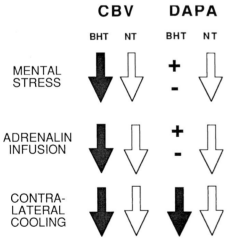

Figure 116. The reaction of capillary blood cell velocity (CBV) and digital arterial pulse amplitude (DAPA) to different stress stimuli studied in borderline hypertensive patients (BHT) and normotensive controls (NT). CBV was equally influenced in the two groups, while in the BHT patients DAPA did not show any reaction to mental stress and adrenal infusion, only to contralateral cooling.

Influence of Hypertension on CBV

The influence of sympatho-adrenal stimulation on skin microvascular dynamics has been studied in a group of patients with borderline hypertension (BHT; BP: 153/88 mmHg) and controls (BP: 123/68 mmHg) (14). Three different tests were used: mental arithmetic stress, infusion of adrenalin, and cooling of the contralateral hand. The nutritional skin circulation was evaluated by measuring the CBV in the finger nailfold capillaries, and the total arterial inflow capacity by plethysmographic recording of the digital arterial pulse amplitude (DAPA).

It was found (**Figure 116**) that during mental stress CBV decreased significantly (p<0.01) in both the BHT patients and the controls, while DAPA decreased (p<0.01) only in the normotensives. A similar pattern in the reaction of CBV and DAPA was seen during infusion of adrenalin (0.8 nmol / kg / min). However, during cooling of the contralateral hand, both DAPA and CBV decreased significantly in both groups.

Comments: The reactivity of the nutritional vascular bed of the skin to different forms of stress stimuli seems to be similar in normotensive and BHT patients. On the other hand, the total arterial inflow to the fingers appears to react much less to stress stimuli in BHT patients than in controls, which may indicate functional or structural changes of the finger arteries or arterioles.

The reaction of DAPA and CBV to contralateral cooling and mental stress has also been studied in a few (n=6) patients with established hypertension (BP: 170/103 mmHg) (6). Quite different patterns of reactivity were seen during contralateral cooling. In some patients there was a marked *increase* of DAPA, while CBV was almost unchanged (**Figure 117**). In other patients, the reversed reaction could be seen. This was the case despite a marked and similiar increase in both systolic and diastolic

Figure 117. Simultaneous recording of total skin circulation by laser Doppler flux and capillary blood cell velocity in a finger of a 35-year-old woman with hypertension. During an arithmetic stress test, the laser Doppler value increased fourfold, while no reaction was seen in the capillary circulation. This demonstrates the discrepancy in reaction that sometimes can be seen between total skin blood flow and capillary circulation during certain circumstances.

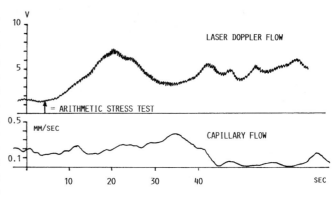

pressure during the stress stimuli in all patients studied.

It could be concluded that individual patients with established essential hypertension may have quite different reactivity in the total and nutritional skin circulation of fingers, so that from this point of view they are a heterogeneous group (6).

Hereditary Teleangiectasia (Rendu-Osler-Weber)

It may be difficult to distinguish between Rendu-Osler-Weber's disease and teleangiectatic form of scleroderma (21). **Figure 118** shows pictures of two patients with similarly looking teleangiectasia of lips and tongue. Both consulted otolaryngologists for repeated epistaxis. Clinically the diagnosis of Osler's disease was made in both patients. Capillaroscopy allowed a correct diagnosis. Indeed, the first patient suffered from the hereditary condition with a fundamentally different prognosis and the second from progressive systemic sclerosis, a diagnosis confirmed during the following years. Proximal scleroderma, severe Raynaud's phenomenon, sclerodactyly and finger tip ulcerations developed in this second patient.

Capillaroscopic images of both patients after application of NaF are shown in **Figure 119** (12). In the first case, the capillary pattern was normal with exception of a well defined convo-

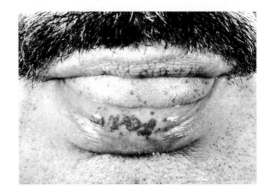
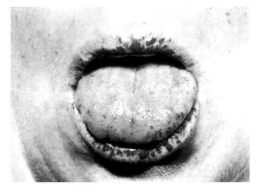

Figure 118. Differential diagnosis between Osler's disease and teleangiectatic form of scleroderma may be difficult. Capillaroscopy allows an accurate differentiation (see Figure 119).
Above: Teleangiectasias of a patient with Osler's disease.
Below: Teleangiectasias of a patient with progressive systemic sclerosis.

Miscellaneous Disorders

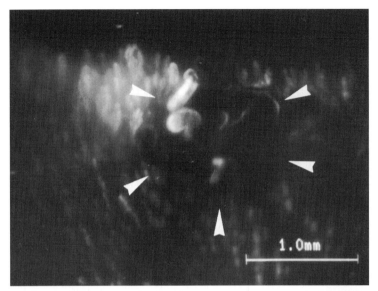

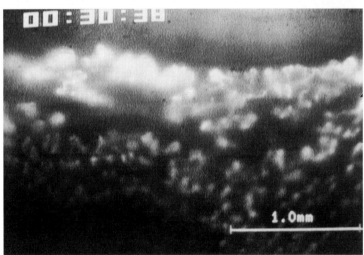

Figure 119.
Above: Osler's nodule near the nailfold consisting of giant and meandering microvessels. The convolute is only partially filled by NaF and embedded in normal capillaries (same patient as in Figure 118a).
Below: Typical microangiopathy speaking in favor of collagen vascular disease (same patient as in Figure 118b).

lute of tortuous megacapillaries. Typical scleroderma-like changes were observed in the patient with progressive systemic sclerosis. Enlarged capillaries, loss of microvessels and increased transcapillary diffusion of NaF could be demonstrated.

The morphological findings in Osler's disease were confirmed in three additional patients (12). Identical images were obtained previously (5). The maximal diameter of the megacapillaries contained in the Osler's nodules reached 150 µm (12).

Flow velocity was decreased in the enlarged microvessels. In some huge capillary loops, microvascular flow was bidirectional (**Figure 120**). After a certain time, the flow direction changed after a flow stop (12). Since the pre- and postcapillary vessels are not visualized by intravital microscopy the exact mechanism of bidirectional capillary flow remains obscure.

Chapter 2.8

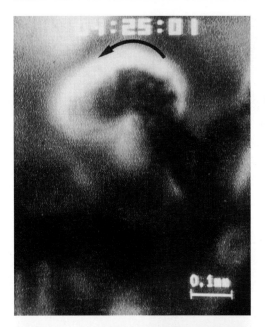

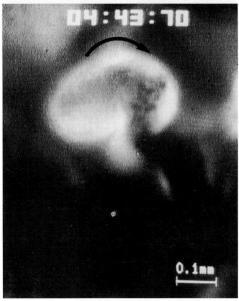

Figure 120. Giant capillary within an Osler's nodule (high magnification). Enhanced contrast for the slowly moving erythrocytes is provided by NaF. The arrows indicate the flow direction, which frequently inversed in this enlarged microvessel.

The capillaroscopic findings in hereditary teleangiectasia Rendu-Osler-Weber are so characteristic that they confirm or delete the diagnosis. A cluster of huge capillaries is embedded in a field of normal microvessels. The enlarged and tortuous capillaries may exhibit pathologic hemodynamics with repeated reversal of flow direction.

Cold Injury

Frostbite damages small arteries, arterioles, capillaries and veins as has been demonstrated in animal experiments (10). Besides vascular occlusions which have been demonstrated in larger human vessels by arteriography (19), cold induced vasospastic changes play an important role (10).

In four patients, capillaroscopy with and without the use of the fluorescent tracer NaF has been performed 1–44 days after cold injury (1). All four exposed their hands and fingers to arctic temperatures when they performed cross-country skiing or mountain climbing. The fingers showed bluish discoloration and formation of blisters. In two patients finger tip necrosis developed.

At capillaroscopy skin transparency was reduced because of edema. Where the local conditions permitted the nailfold and the dorsum of one or several fingers were studied (1). Capillaroscopy without NaF injection was difficult to interpret. Visualization of skin microvessels improved considerably after application of the fluorescent dye.

Fluorescent videomicroscopy revealed areas without perfusion (1). In the example of **Figure 121**, a reduced number of capillaries was filled at the dorsum of the fingers. The depicted groups appeared as islets within dark nonperfused areas. Probably, most capillaries within the dark, nonfluorescent parts were obliterated although prolonged microvascular stasis cannot be ruled out by fluorescence videomicroscopy. Both phenomena, stasis and occlusion, have been demonstrated experimentally (10). In two of the four patients more than 12 s elapsed be-

Miscellaneous Disorders

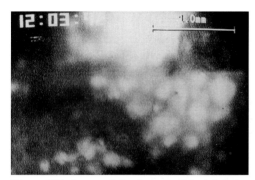

Figure 121. Image of the dorsum of the left index finger after cross-country skiing at very cold temperature. Frostbite caused blister formation. After NaF injection, only some areas are perfused (bright fluorescing spots). Skin transparency is reduced because of edema. Without the application of fluorescent dyes, it is almost impossible to recognize any capillaries.

tween filling of the first and last capillaries (1). Spastic changes at the level of the precapillary vessels or reversible stasis of red cells is probably responsible for this observation.

Fluorescent light intensity was increased around the still perfused microvessels. NaF diffused through the capillary wall in enhanced amounts indicating partial breakdown of the diffusion barriers. Pericapillary halos were never sharply delineated. In one particular patient increased dye passage through the outer halo border and cloud-like dye accumulation were documented (**Figure 122**). The image resembles the findings in progressive systemic sclerosis. Increased permeability of microvessels after cold injury was also described in animal experiments (10). Cold injury to skin microvessels is a good example for the fact that noxious stimuli of different nature may induce similar microvascular changes.

In summary, cold injury elicits dramatic microvascular damage including spastic changes, stasis of erythrocytes in capillary loops, microvascular occlusions and increased permeability of still perfused loops. It is not known whether necrosis developing late after frostbite (19) results from microcirculatory failure or from the participation of larger vessels.

Acrodermatitis chronica atrophicans (ACA) Pick-Herxheimer

The most common cause for local edema and cyanotic discoloration of the lower extremity is acute or chronic venous incompetens (CVI). However, one disease that can produce similar symptoms as CVI is *acrodermatitis chronica atrophicans* (ACA) Pick-Herxheimer, a disease caused by the spirochete *Borrelia burgdorferi*. The typical symptom of ACA is inflammatory

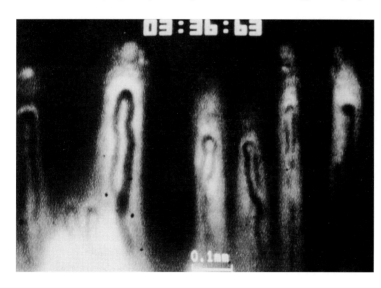

Figure 122. Nailfold capillaries after mild frostbite. The diffusion barrier for NaF at the outer halo border is abolished in part. The dye accumulates in "cloud"-like areas.

151

Figure 123. Microphoto of the skin microvascular bed in a patient with acrodermatitis chronica atrophicans Herxheimer.
Left: In the affected leg the capillaries are seen as small dark dots, and because of the skin atrophy, the subpapillary vascular plexus is prominent and dilated.
Right: On the contralateral leg the vascular plexus cannot be visualized.

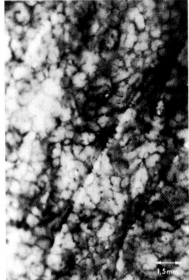 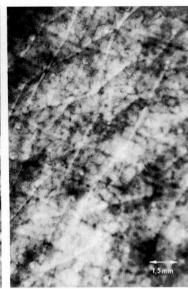

lesions, localized in one or several parts of the extremities. If untreated, the inflammation may persist for years but is gradually replaced by atrophy. In the inflammatory stage, the skin shows a cyanotic discoloration.

Vital capillaroscopy often reveals a clear picture of atrophy with a prominant and dilated subpapillary venular plexus (**Figure 123**) (3, 7). The capillaries are seldom affected. If the affection is localized to the lower leg, it is easily understood that the symptoms can be mistaken for CVI. It has been shown that these patients have a significant increase in the blood flow of the foot and calf region, both compared to the contralateral leg of the patients and to healthy, matched controls (3). The skin temperature is often significantly increased, and the venous capacity and maximal venous return from the leg may also be enhanced.

Studies in Pregnancy and Preeclampsia

Preeclampsia is a common cause of placental insufficiency and fetal intrauterine growth retardation (4, 8). Both blood viscosity and peripheral vascular resistance have been reported to be increased in these patients, indicating the possibility of impaired capillary circulation. Therefore, nailfold skin capillary blood cell velocity (CBV) was measured in 14 healthy pregnant women and 12 preeclamptic patients (16). No difference was found between resting CBV in the preeclamptic group (median 0.58 mm/s) and in the healthy controls (0.52 mm/s). As the plasma expander dextran is said to decrease blood viscosity and increase the circulating blood volume thus improving blood flow, the effect on capillary circulation in these patients was also studied. Following infusion of dextran-70, the CBV in the preeclamptic patients increased by 154% compared to preinfusion values ($p<0.05$). These results show that increasing the plasma volume in patients with preeclampsia may improve the nutritional circulation of tissues. Whether the circulation is also increased in the placenta and other organs is, of course, not possible to evaluate from these results.

The reactivity of the skin microcirculation was also studied in women with normal pregnancy and in a group of patients with preeclampsia (17). It was found that vasomotion, assessed by the rhythmic variation of CBV, was similar in all groups investigated regarding frequency (3–10 cycles/m) and amplitude (0.01–

0.23 mm/s). In healthy control subjects, basal CBV was positively correlated with the amplitude of the individual velocity fluctuations. The CBV response to venous occlusion was significantly reduced ($p<0.05$) in preeclampsia compared to normal pregnancies and nonpregnant controls. These findings indicate that an impaired veno-arteriolar reflex may contribute to the edema formation often seen in patients with preeclampsia.

Sympathetic Dystrophies

Dystrophy of the sympathetic nerves in limbs may be caused by trauma (20). However, other disorders like myocardial infarction, cerebral vascular disease, and cervical osteochondrosis may also give rise to a similar syndrome (9). The effect on the skin microcirculation was studied in 12 patients with sympathetic dystrophies secondary to trauma or other diseases. The finger nailfold capillary blood cell velocity (CBV) was measured. Laser Doppler fluxmetry (LDF) was also used to provide an index of skin microcirculation in the vessels in addition to the superficial capillaries. Both the CBV and LDF values were significantly lower in the patients compared to healthy controls ($p<0.05$), despite the skin temperature being the same in both groups. During cooling of the contralateral hand, CBV and LDF decreased markedly (22–60%) in the control group, but no such decrease could be seen in the patients (0–13%). The veni-vasomotor reflex normally seen when lowering the hand was also almost completely absent in the patient group (7%) compared to the controls (42%). These results indicate that the vasomotor reflex responses are damaged in patients with sympathetic dystrophies and may well explain some of the typical features of the syndrome, for example, the edema. In another study of the same group, it was found that also in the nonaffected hand of these patients the response to contralateral cooling is significantly disturbed, indicating that there is also a malfunction of the central nervous control of the skin microcirculation in these patients (18).

Other Disorders

The morphology and circulation in the skin capillaries have also been studied in a number of other diseases. It could be mentioned that rather marked changes of the morphological pattern can be seen, for example, in patients with *schizophrenia*. Maricq has described this phenomenon in a number of papers (13). By using a specific plexus visualization score (PVS), it has been found that schizophrenic patients have a much more prominent subpapillary vascular plexus than control subjects, and they much more easily suffer capillary hemorrhages. The reason for the change in nailfold capillary morphology is not fully understood.

Lipowsky et al. have used intravital microscopy for studying capillary hemodynamic in *sickle-cell disease* (11). It was found that the CBV was normal in sickle-cell patients in crisis-free intervals. In contrast, CBV was significantly elevated during the crisis, which is thought to result from compensatory arteriolar dilatation. On the other hand, the postocclusive reactive hyperemia response was reduced in the sickle-cell patients during crisis, which is thought to result from red cell deformation and leucocyte endothelium adhesion during the crisis.

References 2.8

1) Baer, H. U., Baer-Suryadinata, Ch., Segantini, P., Bollinger, A.: Kapillarschäden nach Erfrierungen an den Akren, beurteilt durch die Fluoreszenz-Videomikroskopie. *Schweizerische med. Wschr.* 115, 479–483, 1985.

2) Berglund, G., Ljungman, S., Hartford, M., Wikstrand, J. Aurell, M.: Total, renal and calf muscle vascular resistance in relation to blood pressure. Possible implications for the development of essential hypertension. Milan, Italy: First European Meeting on Hypertension, 29th May–1st June, 1983. (abstract)

3) Bollinger, A.: *Funktionelle Angiologie.* Thieme, Stuttgart, 1979.

4) Buchan, P. C.: Preeclampsia. A hyperviscosity syndrome. *Am J. Obst. Gyn.* 112, 111–112, 1982.
5) Davis, M. J., Lawler, J. C.: The capillary circulation of the skin. *Arch. Dermatol.* 77, 690–703, 1958.
6) Fagrell, B.: Microcirculatory methods for the clinical assessment of hypertension, hypotension, and ischemia. *Ann. Biomed. Eng.* 14;163–173, 1986.
7) Fagrell, B., Stiernstedt, G., Östergren, J.: Acrodermatitis chronica atrophicans herxheimer can often mimic a peripheral vascular disorder. *Acta. Med. Scand.* 220, 485–488, 1986.
8) Gallery, E. D. M., Hunyor, S. N., Gyory, A.Z.: Plasma volume contraction: A significant factor in both pregnancy-associated and chronic hypertension in pregnancy. *Quar. J. Med.* 192, 593–602, 1979
9) Kozin, F., McCarty, D. J., Sims, J., Genant, H.: The reflex sympathetic dystrophy syndrome. *Am. J. Med.* 60, 321–331, 1976.
10) Laprell-Moschner, Ch., Endrich, B., Brendel, W., Messmer, K.: A model for studies of the microcirculation during chronic exposure to cold. *Microvasc. Res.* 26, 271, 1983.
11) Lipowsky, H. H., Sheikh, N. U., Katz, D. M.: Intravital microscopy of capillary hemodynamics in sickle cell disease. *J. Clin. Invest.* 80, 117–127, 1986.
12) Maire, R., Schnewlin, G., Bollinger, A.: Videomikroskopische Untersuchungen von Teleangiektasien bei Morbus Osler und Sklerodermie. *Schweiz. med. Wschr.* 116, 335–338, 1986.
13) Maricq, H. R.: Capillary fragility and visualization of subpapillary plexus in the nailfold of schizophrenic patients. *Bibl. Anat.* 10, 389–397, 1968.
14) Östergren, J., Fagrell, B., de Faire, U., Hjemdahl, P., Kahan, T.: Skin microcirculation in borderline hypertensive patients and controls during sympatho-adrenal activation. XIIIth World Congress, International Union of Angiology, July, 1983. (Abstract).
15) Rosén, L., Östergren, J., Fagrell, B., Stranden, E.: Skin microvascular circulation in the sympathetic dystrophies evaluated by video photometric capillaroscopy and laer Doppler fluxmetry. *Eur. J. clin. Invest.* 18, 305–308, 1988.
16) Rosén, L., Östergren, J., Fagrell, B., Stranden, E.: Skin capillary blood cell velocity in preeclampsia. The effect of plasma expansion. *Int. J. Microcirc.: Clin. Exp.* 8, 237–244, 1989.
17) Rosén, L., Östergren, J., Fagrell, B., Stranden, E.: Mechanisms for edema formation in pregnancy and preeclampsia as evaluated skin capillary dynamics. *Int. J. Microcirc.: Clin. Exp.*, in print.
18) Rosén, L., Östergren, J., Roald, O. K., Stranden, E., Fagrell, B.: Bilateral involvement and the effect of sympathetic blockade on skin microcirculation in the sympathetic dystrophies. *Microvasc. Res.* 37, 289–297, 1989.
19) Segantini, P.: Angiologische Aspekte der lokalen Erfrierung. *Z. Unfallmed. Berufskr.* 73, 171–174, 1980.
20) Sudeck, P.: Über die acute entzundliche Knochenatrophie. *Arch. Klin. Chir.* 62, 147–156, 1900.
21) Winterbauer, R. H.: Multiple telangiectasia. Raynaud's phenomenon, sclerodactyly and subcutaneous calcinosis: A syndrome mimicking hereditary hemorrhagic telangiectasia. *Bull. Johns Hopk. Hosp.* 114, 361–383, 1964.
22) Zweifler, A. J., Nicholls, G.: Diminished finger volume pulse in borderline hypertension: Evidence for early structural vascular abnormality. *Am. Heart. J.* 104, 812–815, 1982.

3

CONTROL OF THERAPY

3.1 Pharmacological Agents

Several pharmacological agents have a strong effect on skin microcirculation. The effect of a few of these on CBV have been studied during recent years, and a few of these studies will be reviewed.

Calcium Antagonists

The calcium antagonist nifedipine has a marked vasodilatory effect on skin blood vessels (6, 7). The effect of this substance on capillary blood flow in the nailfold has been studied in 8 healthy controls. The subjects were given sublingually a capsule containing 10 mg of nifedipine or placebo. The capsule was crushed in the mouth, and the content was absorbed through the mucous membrane of the mouth. Recordings of CBV were performed every other minute for 20 minutes after administration; skin temperature, digital arterial pulse amplitude (DAPA), and heart rate were also recorded at 2-minute intervals. Mean rCBV before application of the capsule was approximately equal in both groups (0.56 mm/s and 0.54 mm/s, respectively). As can be seen in **Figure 124**, there was a slight (n.s.) decrease of rCBV after application of placebo, but a significant (p<0.01) increase in rCBV after nifedipine. DAPA increased less (n.s.) on nifedipine.

Comments: The increase in CBV was achieved in spite of any significant increase in

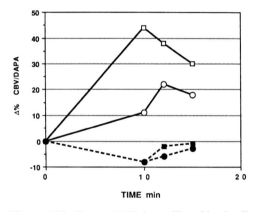

Figure 124. Change (Δ%) in capillary blood cell velocity (CBV) and digital arterial pulse amplitude (DAPA) after sublinguinal application of nifedipin (nif), or placebo (pl). Nifedipine significantly (p<0.01) increased CBV but affected the total skin blood flow (DAPA) only to a minor degree (n.s.). □ = Δ% CBV/nif; ○ = Δ% DAPA/nif; ■ = Δ% CVB/pl; ● = Δ% DAPA/pl.

skin temperature or total arterial inflow to the region. This suggests that nifedipine has a more prominent effect on nutritional skin capillary flow than on thermoregulatory flow, which seems to be separately regulated (1). The combination of macro- and microcirculatory measurements in the skin is therefore of great importance for evaluating the effect of drugs in different vascular compartments of the skin microcirculation.

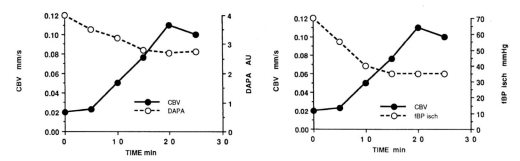

Figure 125. The effect of sublingual application of nifedipine (time 0) on capillary blood cell velocity (CBV), digital arterial pulse amplitude (DAPA), and systolic blood pressure (fBP) in an ischemic finger of a patient with obliteration of the brachial artery of the arm. As can be seen, CBV increased about fourfold despite a marked decrease of both fBP and DAPA! This shows that the nutritional blood flow may increase dramatically in an ischemic area despite even a *decrease* of the total circulation of the region.

In one patient with a thrombotic occlusion of the left brachial artery, the acute effect of nifedipin was also studied (**Figure 125**). This was done to investigate the effect of the substance in one region with a reduced, and in one with a normal, arterial circulation. Ten to 15 min after sublingual application of nifedine, both the systemic and digital blood pressure decreased by 35 mmHg (**Figure 125**). At the same time, DAPA decreased by 30%, but nevertheless CVB increased by 400%!

This clearly shows that a vasodilator may have a positive effect on the nutritional skin circulation in ischemic areas, even though the total circulation of the area is reduced (2). This is of great importance in clinical practice, as it has been seriously questioned if vasodilators can ever have a positive effect in regions with a reduced arterial blood flow.

Prostanoids

The effect of prostaglandins on the nutritional skin microcirculation was studied in 13 patients with rest pain and skin necrosis, waiting for lower leg amputation (4). The PGE_1 was administered as a continuous infusion in a subclavia catheter for three days. The microcirculation of the affected foot was evaluated by SBP and the effect on the skin circulation by vital capil-

laroscopy. The structural changes of the skin capillaries were classified according to the 7-point scale presented on page 64.

SBP did not change during the treatment (**Figure 126**). Nevertheless, the capillary score did improve in eight of the 13 patients—sometimes dramatically (**Figure 126**). Seven patients noted pain relief lasting from a few days up to more than 3 weeks. A good correlation was found between clinical improvement of symptoms and improvement in capillary score, and in spite of no improvement of the total circulation to the area, two patients healed completely after treatment.

Comments: Also this study indicates that a vasoactive drug (PGE_1) may improve the skin microcirculation without any noticeable effect on the macrocirculation.

β-blockers

Disturbance of the peripheral circulation is a clinical problem during antihypertensive treatment with some β-adrenoreceptor blocking agents. Vasospastic phenomenon, claudication, and even gangrene of the skin (5) have been associated with betablocking therapy. The effect of a β-blocking agent (pindolol) on capillary

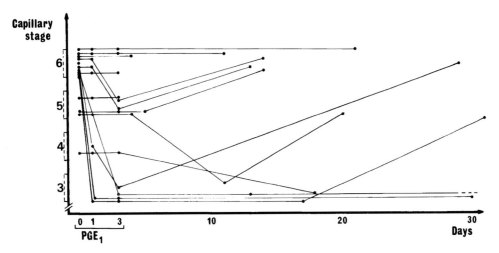

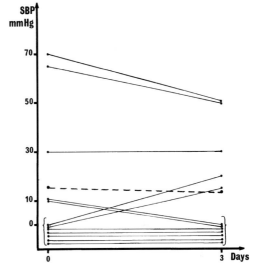

Figure 126. The total arterial circulation as evaluated by the systolic blood pressure of the toe (SBP) and the skin nutritional circulation (Capillary stage) were evaluated in 13 patients with critical limb ischemia and gangrene before and during 3 days of treatment with PGE$_1$. In spite of no change of SBP during the PGE$_1$ infusion (mean value is indicated by the dashed line), the capillary stage improved in most of the patients during or after infusion. In two patients, the capillaries became completely filled with blood, and these patients also healed their gangrene within 8 weeks after treatment.

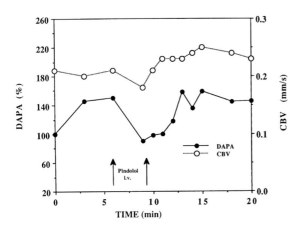

Figure 127. The effect ($\bar{x} \pm SD$) of 1 mg pindolol (i.v.) on digital arterial pulse amplitude (DAPA) and capillary blood cell velocity (CBV) in fingers of 5 healthy subjects. A decrease can be seen in both DAPA and CBV during the injection, which is caused by a sympathetic reflex. After infusion DAPA and CBV return to preinfusion values.

blood cell velocity (CBV) was studied in five healthy male subjects (26–40 yrs) (3). All had normal finger blood pressures. CBV was slightly reduced during injection of 1 mg of pindolol intravenously (**Figure 127**). This decrease in CBV is probably explained by the reduced arterial inflow as evaluated by a decrease of the digital arterial pulse amplitude (DAPA) in the finger. Following the injection, CBV showed a small, nonsignificant increase, while DAPA was unchanged (**Figure 127**). The peak CBV during postocclusive reactive hyperemia after a 1-minute arterial occlusion was also the same before and after pindolol. The results indicate that pindolol in healthy young subjects does not reduce skin capillary blood cell velocity during resting conditions. Neither does the ability to produce maximal, or near-maximal vasodilatation, seem to be impaired after administration of i.v. pindolol. The role of the intrinsic sympatho-mimetic effect (ISA) of pindolol on β_2-adrenoreceptors must be decided from further studies comparing pindolol with β-adrenoreceptor blockers without ISA.

References 3.1

1) Coffman, J. D.: Total and nutritional blood flow in the finger. *Clin. Sci.* 42, 243–250, 1972.
2) Fagrell, B.: Are vasodiling substances really bad for patients with ischemic leg symptoms? In: *Conservative Therapy of Arterial Occlusive Disease.* Georg Thieme Verlag, Stuttgart. Ed. G. Trübestein, pp. 64–67, 1986.
3) Fagrell, B., Östergren, J.: Effect of intravenously administered pindolol on skin capillary blood cell velocity in fingers. *Br. J. clin. Pharmac.* 13, 233S–235S, 1982.
4) Fagrell, B., Lundberg, G., Olsson, A.G., Östergren, J.: PGE_1 treatment of severe skin ischemia in patients with peripheral arterial insufficiency–The effect on skin microcirculation. *VASA* 15, 56–60, 1986.
5) Gokal, R., Dorner, T. L., Ledingham, J. G. G.: Peripheral skin necrosis complicating β-blockade. *Br. Med. J.* 2, 721–722, 1979.
6) Pola, P., Savi, L.: Peripheral vascular dynamics studied by calcium ion inhibition. *Angiology* 29, 506–519, 1978.
7) Östergren, J., Fagrell, B.: Videophotometric capillaroscopy for evaluating drug effects on skin microcirculation–A double-blind study with nifedipine. *Clin. Phys.* 4, 169–176, 1984.

3.2 Interventional Therapy

Reconstructive Vascular Surgery

Improvement of Capillary Morphology

The structure of the nutritional skin capillaries changes dramatically in areas of ischemia (see page 63ff.). If the macrocirculation to the ischemic area improves, the structure and blood filling of the nutritional capillaries would also improve. In order to test this the structure of the nutritional capillaries were investigated before and after femoro-popliteal saphenous vein by pass operations in eight legs with ischemic rest pain or ulcerations (3). The skin nutritional circulation of the feet was evaluated by the capillary classification shown in **Figure 8** (page 7). The macrocirculation was evaluated by the digital blood pressure (SBP). Investigations were preformed 1 week before, 1–2 and 5–6 weeks after the operation.

Following the reconstructive procedure, intraoperative basal graft blood flow rate was increased ($p<0.01$) from 153 ml/min to 237 ml/min. After the operation, the mean SBP increased to almost twice the value recorded before the operation ($p<0.05$). In the contralateral, unoperated leg there was no change in SBP during the 6-week observation period. The nutritional skin circulation improved somewhat, though not significantly, during the first 2 weeks after operation, and in one patient there was even a deterioration of the nutritional vascular bed. However, after 6 weeks, all patients had improved microscopically ($p<0.05$) from 4.5 to 2.3 units in mean capillary stage (**Figure 128**). In one patient the SBP decreased although the nutritional circulation was improved and the patient was relieved of pain. In one patient the total circulation of the foot improved, but in spite of this the patient deteriorated microscopically and also developed blisters followed by necrotic areas on several toes. These two examples show that there may be a discrepancy between the macro- and microcirculation in a certain skin region, making it difficult to predict what will happen in these two vascular compartments when the total blood flow is suddenly increased. Capillaroscopy seems to give valuable information regarding the nutritional status of ischemic areas also after reconstructive surgery.

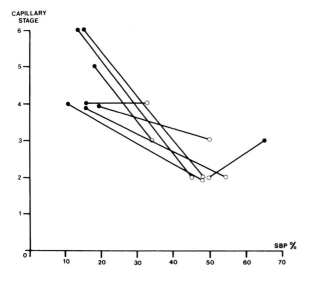

Figure 128. Capillary stage and systolic blood pressure of the big toe expressed as percent of the arm blood pressure (SBP%) in patients with PAOD, before (●) and after (○) femoro-popliteal reconstructive vascular surgery. In all but one patient, the blood pressure increased after the operation, and in all but one patient the capillary stage also improved.

Improvement of Capillary Blood Cell Velocity

Schwartz et al. (6) studied the effect of reconstructive femoro-popliteal bypass surgery on the local skin capillary circulation of the toes. Despite a significant increase in the total arterial circulation of the foot, there was no improvement of the capillary circulation. The reason for this is unclear, but it may be explained by the rather short time (1 week) between the operation and the postoperative investigation. As was seen in the study of morphology changes after the operation described above, no significant improvement was noticed 2 weeks after operation, but after 6 weeks a significant improvement was seen. It has also been suggested that restoration of the reactivity of the precapillary sphincters may require up to 2 months following reconstructive surgery (7).

Catheter Therapy

Similar to the findings after reconstructive arterial surgery, blood flow to the foot increases considerably after successful percutaneous transluminal angioplasty (PTA), local thrombolysis with streptokinase or urokinase, and thrombectomy by catheters. Intermittent claudication, rest pain, or incipient gangrene may be improved or cured.

The improvement of macrovascular hemodynamics, documented by systolic ankle or toe pressure measurements or other adequate techniques, is accompanied by changes of capillaroscopic findings outlined above. A study using fluorescence video microscopy has been performed to control the success of PTA. The main results are described on pages 73 and 74. During postischemic hyperemia, transcapillary diffusion of NaF at the forefoot is still more enhanced than before relieving ischemia by PTA. Postischemic edema often develops during this period. One month after successful catheter treatment, the interstitial accumulation of the small fluorescent solute NaF has dropped to almost normal values.

Sympathetic Blockade

It has been disputed that lumbal sympathetic blockade (LSB) is of benefit to patients with ischemic rest pain and skin necrosis from severe PAOD of the lower limb (5, 8, 9). No study has convincingly shown that the total arterial circulation of the ischemic area is improved by LSB, which shows that the clinical effect on the microcirculation of the ischemic area cannot be evaluated objectively with macrocirculatory methods. Therefore, the effect of LSB on the structure of the nutritional capillaries of ischemic skin areas was evaluated by capillaroscopy in 10 patients suffering from ischemic rest pain and trophic ulcers of the foot (2). The total circulation of the region was evaluated by systolic blood pressure measurement of the big toe (SBP), expressed as a percentage of the arm blood pressure (SBP%). The nutritional capillaries of the dorsum of the toes were studied according to the technique described on page 64, using the 7-stage classification.

All patients had a systolic toe blood pressure of less that 20 mmHg in the supine position before LSB, and it did not improve by the procedure. The mean SBP% of the affected foot was $8.1 \pm 3.2\%$ before, and $8.9 \pm 3\%$ 3 days after LSB had been performed. The patients were followed up to 3 weeks after LSB, and there was no change of the SBP% during this period. However, the nutritional microcirculation successively improved in seven of the investigated patients, and concomitantly the clinical signs like rest pain and ischemic ulcers also improved. In those patients in whom deterioration of the capillary circulation could be seen, no improvement of the clinical status occured (**Figure 129**).

Comments: It has been questioned whether LSB can be an alternative treatment for ischemic rest pain and necrosis in patients with PAOD. The best results seem to be achieved in patients with proximal single stenosis (1). The microscopic improvement noticed by capillaroscopy was not reflected by an improved arterial inflow to the area as evaluated by SBP%. This discrepancy may be explain by a

Interventional Therapy

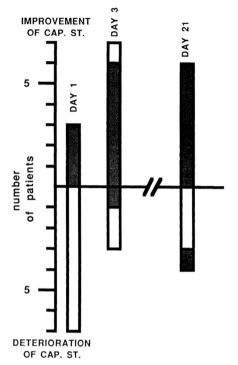

Figure 129. Improvement or deterioration of the capillary stage in 10 patients, 1, 3 and 21 days after lumbal sympathetic blockade. The shaded parts of the columns indicate patients who improved clinically; the white parts reflect those who did not show any clinical improvement. Twenty-one days after the operation full agreement was seen between the capillary and clinical improvement in all but one patient.

very peripheral effect of the sympathetic block. If it reduces the resistance of the precapillary arterioles, distally to the arteriovenous anastomoses in the ischemic skin area (which are especially numerous in the digits), blood may be transformed from these nonnutritional vessels into the nutritional capillaries. This may be the reason why a positive clinical effect of LSB can be recorded despite no measurable improvement of the total arterial circulation of the area. Once again, a discrepancy between the effect on macro- and microcirculation is demonstrated by this study, and it illustrates the necessity to use microcirculatory methods for recording objectively the clinical effect achieved.

Spinal Cord Stimulation

Epidural electrical spinal cord stimulation (ESES) is a technique that has been accepted as a therapeutic modality for the control of chronic pain. It has been found that this therapy may be successfully used also in patients with ischemic rest pain. Strikingly enough, not only pain relief may be achieved, but also the healing of ischemic ulcers (4), which implies that the nutritional blood flow in the ischemic area is improved. Macrocirculatory methods have been used for objective evaluation of the effect of ESES, but here too all attempts have so far failed. The reason most probably lies, as in the cases of sympathetic blockade, in these techniques not being sensitive enough to evaluate the effect of a therapy on microcirculation. Jacobs et al. (4) recently studied the effect of ESES in 10 patients with severe limb ischemia due to arteriosclerotic disease. Microcirculatory parameters were assest before and after the treatment. The following parameters were studied:

1) Capillary density,

2) Blood cell velocity,

3) Transportation of fluorescent dyes.

After ESES the clinical improvement was confirmed by the microscopic techniques. Capillary density increased ($p<0.001$), and CBV improved from 0.05 mm/s to 0.76 mm/s ($p<0.001$). Also, the appearance time of the fluorescent dye decrease significantly ($p<0.001$) from 72-45 s, but the macrocirculatory method (systolic ankle/arm pressure ratios) did not change at all.

Comments: The results of the present study once again shows that the skin microcirculation of ischemic areas can be significantly improved despite no measurable improvement of the macrocirculation. Treatments of patients with PAOD and ischemic skin lesions should consequently be evaluated by microcirculatory methods in order to objectively prove the clinical effect.

References 3.2

1) Boas, R. A.: Sympathetic blocks in clinical practice. *Int. Anesthes. Clin.* 16, 149–182, 1978.
2) Fagrell, B., McInerney, D., Johansson, H., Juhlin-Dannfelt, A.,, Linde, B., Lundblad, B., Sonnenfeldt, T.: The effect of lumbal sympathetic block on the nutritional circulation of ischemic skin areas in patients with rest pain and gangrene. In: *New Developments in Angiology* Plenum, pp. 1123–1126, 1984.
3) Fagrell, B., Sonnenfeld, T., Cronestrand, R., Lind, M.: The microcirculatory response to reconstructive vascular surgery in patients with severe foot ischemia. *Bibl. Anat.* (Karger) 18, 385–388, 1979.
4) Jacobs, M., Jörning, P., Joshi, S., Kitslaar, P., Slaaf, D., Reneman, R.: Epidural spinal cord electrical stimulation improves microvascular blood flow in severe limb ischemia. *Ann. Surg.* 207, 179–183, 1988.
5) Nielsen, P. E., Bell, G., Augustenborg, G., Paaske-Hanssen, O., Lassen, N. A.: Reduction in distal blood pressure by sympathetic nerve block in patients with occlusive arterial disease. *Cardiovasc. Res.* 7, 577–584, 1973.
6) Schwartz, R. W., Freedman, A. M., Richardson, D. R., Hyde, G. L., Griffen, W. O., Vincent, D. G., Price, M. A.: Capillary blood flow: Videodensitometry in the atherosclerotic patient. *J. Vasc. Surg.* 1, 800–808, 1984.
7) Simeone, F. A., Husni, E. A.: The hyperemia of reconstructive arterial surgery. *Ann. Surg.* 150, 575–585, 1959.
8) Thulesius, O., Gjöres, J. E., Mandaus, L.: Distal blood pressure in vascular occlusion. Influence of sympathetic nerves on callateral blood flow. *Scand. J. clin. Invest. Lab.* (Suppl. 31), 53–58, 1973.
9) Uhrenholdt, A., Dam, W. H., Larsen, O. A., Lassen, N. A., Para et al.: Paradoxical effect on peripheral blood flow after sympathetic blockades in patients with gangrene due to arteriosclerosis obliterans. *Vasc. Surg.* 5, 154–163, 1971.

SUBJECT INDEX

acral necrosis 139
acridyl orange 31
acrocyanosis 117
acrodermatitis chronica atrophicans (ACA) 151
aggregation, erythrocyte 11, 15, 97
albumin, FITC-labeled 53, 54
aldose reductase 78
aminoguanidine 78
amputation levels 69
aneurysmatic dilatation 6
angioplasty, peripheral transluminal 71, 73, 160
ankle 49, 54, 95
ankylosis, of ankle-joint 93
antibodies, anti-DNA 124, 138
aplasia, microlymphatics 109
appearance time 37, 46, 71, 70, 118
arterial occlusive disease 63–76
arteriography 89
arteriolar limb 5
arterioles 46, 68, 71, 161
arteriovenous (AV) 68
asphyxia digitorum 118
atrophie blanche 91, 98–101, 104, 123
autoregulation 73, 80
avascular areas 41, 101, 104, 122, 126, 130

basal laminae 123
basement membranes 77, 78
β-blockers 156
 – pindolol 156
bleomycin 139
blisters 112
blood pressure cuff 4
borderline hypertensive patients (BHT) 147
borrelia burgdorferi 151

calcinosis 124
calcium antagonists 155
candle-light phenomenon 71, 72
CapiFlow® 16, 19
capillaroscopy
 – dynamic, with dyes 31–49
 – dynamic, without dyes 9–27
 – and measurement of tcPo$_2$ 60, 61
 – ordinary 1–9
capillary
 – aneurysmatic dilatation 6
 – aneurysms 135

– blood-filled 64
– configuration 6
– density 5, 79, 85, 104, 161
– diameter 5, 19, 37, 38, 44, 45, 56, 80, 115, 117, 122, 135
– dilatation 94
– distribution 6
– flow stop 116, 125
– giant 122
– of hands and feet 5
– hemorrhages 64, 65
– indistinct 64
– loss of 123
– lymphatic 103, 107, 109, 111
– morphological changes of 63
– morphological classifications 7
– morphological patterns 5
– morphology 79–80
– neoformation 123
– neogenesis 78
– normal structure of 5
– number 43, 48, 99
– nutritional skin 63, 67, 79
– papillary 64
– pressure 82, 95
– skin 64
– small dot/comma-shaped 64
– stage 65
– thrombosis 125, 150
– visible 64
– volume flow 80
capillary blood cell velocity (CBV) 9, 12, 43, 44, 80, 87, 95, 115, 117, 118, 124
– accuracy of measurements 16
– analysis of 13–16
– changes of 67
– computerized system for 16–17
– and ESES 161
– effect of smoking on 26
– in full-term neonates 26–27
– influences of hypertension 147
– improvement of 160
– measurement techniques for 9, 11
– nailfold 67
– pulse components of 19
catheter, therapy 160
choroideal vessels 32
chronic granulocyctic leukemia (CGL) 146
chronic lymphocytic leukemia (CLL) 146
chronic respiratory disease 145

chronic venous imcompetence (CVI) 61, 93–105
circulation
– arterial 63, 65
– disturbance of peripheral 156
– nutritional 63
– nutritional skin 147
– total skin 148
claudication
– and β-blockers 156
– intermittent 71
clearance of radioisotopes 80
clefts, interendothelial 53
cobble-stone aspect 96
cold
– hypersensitivity 116, 122, 124
– injury 150
– provocation 116, 118, 124
collagen type IV 78
collagen vascular disease 71, 121–137
collateral vessels 71
collectors, lymphatic 107
compression bandages 95
computer tomography 114
conjunctiva 8, 79
– bulbar 3
cooling of the contralateral hand 153
cooling procedures 23
connective tissue disease, mixed 116, 121
creatine phosphokinase 137
cross-correlation method 15
cryoglobulinemia 124
cryoproteinemia 139

densitometry 39–44, 58, 88, 99, 122
– curves 41, 42, 48, 83
– evaluation 43
– rectangular areas 41
– of several capillaries 41
– of single capillaries 40, 41
– window 42
dermatomyositis 124, 137
dermatosclerotic areas 101
dextran, FITC-labeled 31, 54–57, 101, 102, 107
dextra-70 145
diabetes 77–92, 137
– late complications 81
diffusion
– asymmetrical transcapillary 130
– barriers 85, 88, 125

Subject Index

– distance 61
– interstitial 47, 84, 98, 101, 125, 130
– normal 46
– oxygen 73
– reproducibility of 49
– transcapillary 41, 43, 47, 48, 61, 71, 72, 82, 84, 98, 101, 104, 116, 125, 126, 131
digital arterial pulse amplitude (DAPA) 147
dual-windows technique 14, 15
duplex scanning 89
"dwarf hat" formation 134
dyes 31–34, 54
– and allergic phenomena 31
– fluoresent 31, 69
– transportation of, in ESES 161
dystrophy, sympathetic 153

edema 73, 93, 94, 103, 150
– cardiac 107
– indurated 104
– lymphatic 105, 107
– nephrotic 107
– postischemic 160
electric spinal cord stimulation (ESES) 161
elephantiasis 107
embolism 118
endangiitis obliterans 118
endothelial cells 53, 73, 78, 123
eosinophilic fasciitis 137
erysipelata 112, 113
erythrocyte aggregates 11, 15
erythrocyte column 44
esophageal dysmotility 124

Fåhraeus-Lindqvist effect 45
fibrin layers, pericapillary 99
filaments, anchoring 53
filters
– blue 2, 9, 35
– fluorescence 32
– green 9
– heat 35
– heat-absorbing 2
– "pol-cube" 35
filtration rate 73
finger holder 11
finger nailfold capillaries 11
flow distribution, microvascular 32, 46, 130
flow
– pattern 118
– reversal 118, 149
flow-motion activity 20, 25, 68
fluorescence fading 43
fluorescence microscope 34
– filters 35
– support 35

fluorescence video microscopy 31–52
– and capillary aneurysms 137
– data processing 37–44
– image enhancement 37
– procedure 36–37
– system for 34–36
fluorescent tracers 31–34
FITC-HA fluorescein (isothiocyanat-human albumin) 5
FITC-labeled
– albumin 53, 54
– dextran 53, 54, 56, 58, 101, 102, 107
flux 60
– motion 69
flying spot technique 14
foot
– diabetic 77, 78
– dorsum 49, 63, 69, 79, 85, 107
frame-to-frame analysis 13
frostbite 150

gangrene 71, 87, 88, 156
– digital 139
gingiva 3, 8
glass cylinder, transparent 61
glomeruli 94
glucose 78
glycosylation of proteins 78, 88

halo
– of abnormal shape 125
– border 85
– diameter 38, 44, 45, 95, 97, 134
– pericapillary 47, 48, 84, 85, 94, 95, 103, 116, 130, 134, 135
HbA$_{1C}$ 80, 87
hematocrit
– age-related drop in neonates 27
– and primary polycythemia 144
– and CBV 25
– relative 24
– in skin 27
– variations 24
– zero 24
hematological disorders 144–146
hemoconcentration 98
hemodilution 144
– isovolemic 145
hemodynamics, microvascular 77, 89
homogeneity 42
hyperemia
– reactive 46, 61, 79, 80, 81, 146
– postischemic 73
hyperemic reaction 21
hyperglycemia 77, 78
hyperpigmentation 93
hyperglasia 111
– of arterioles 123
hypertension 147

– influence on CBV 147
hypotensive shock 32, 34

illumination 2
image analysis 56, 58
image analysis system 37
image-shearing monitors 37, 56
immobilization 11
indocyanine green (ICG) 31, 32, 36, 38, 46, 125, 135
– technique 44
infarction, cutaneous 99
infection 87, 88
– streptococci 112
infrared portion of spectrum 32
insufficiency
– perforators 93
– valvular 93, 103, 109
– placental 152
insulin 80, 84
interleukin-1 78
interstitial
– fluid 99, 102, 107, 111
– space 48, 53, 55, 58, 84, 126
interventional therapy 159–161
intravital microscopy 21, 31
irradiation 113
ischemia 61, 63–76
– hand and fingers 118, 121
– microvascular 99
– nutritional skin capillaries 159
– peripheral 69, 71, 87
lamp
– mercury vapor 34
– Xenon 35
laser Doppler 12, 35, 61, 69
– and blood cell flux 12
– probes 10
– fluxmetry (LDF) 67, 69, 81, 148, 153
leg 4, 8
leucocytes 15, 73
leukemia 144, 145
light intensities 39
– fluorescent 39, 85
– gradients 84
lip 3, 8, 148
lumbal sympathetic blockade 160, 161
lupus erythematosus 137
lymphatics, initial 53
lymphedema 56, 107, 114
– congenital (Nonne-Milroy) 108, 114
– differential diagnosis of 113
– primary, sporadic 109, 114
– postmastectomy 113
– secondary 113
– venous incompetence 102, 114
lymph nodes 107, 109
– tumor invasion of 113

Subject Index

lymphography
 – conventional 107, 109
 – indirect 101, 107

macroangiopathy, diabetic 77, 88
macromolecules 53
macrophage receptor 78
malum perforans 88
magnetic resonance 114
magnification 2, 11, 15
megacapillaries 101, 149
mental arithmetic stress test 147, 148
metal bracket 11
microaneurysm 77, 82, 132, 137
microangiopathy
 – diabetic 61, 77, 80, 89
 – functional 89
 – lymphatic 99, 102, 112
 – prognostic value of 124
 – scleroderma 122
 – venous disease 93–106
microlymphatics
 – aplasia 108
 – diameter of 53, 109
 – dye extension 56, 111
 – ectasia 109
 – mesh 53
 – networks 53, 55, 102
 – permeability 56, 103, 111
 – obliteration 102, 112
 – venous disease 102
microlymphography, fluorescence 53–58, 101, 107, 111
micromanipulator 55
microneedle 54
micropools 6
microscope 1, 34
 – IREM-EB-XH 5P/L 10
 – lamp 2, 34, 35
 – Leitz Laborlux 12 ME D 10
 – photomacrography system 1
 – stand 10
 – suspension of 2
 – systems for CBV 9
 – widefield system 1
 – Wild-Leitz 3M® 1, 2
microsyringe 54
microthrombosis 98, 130
microtrauma 126
microvessels, loss of 82
migraine 115
miniature cuff 12
Müller, Otfried 121
muscle pump 93
myo-inositol 78
myxedema 107

Na-fluorescein (NaF) 31, 32, 36, 38, 41, 46–50, 71, 82, 95, 114, 125–134, 149
 – appearance of 46, 69

 – coupling 48, 88
 – plasma 88
 – use of 125
nailfold
 – finger 4
 – capillaries 4, 5, 49, 88, 115, 121, 122, 149
nephropathy 85
neuropathy 77, 81, 85, 88
nifedipine 155, 156
Nonne-Milroy's Disease 108
normotensive controls (NT) 147

occlusion
 – duration 20
 – one-minute arterial 21
 – venous 21, 80
 – femoral artery 71
 – microvascular 76, 98
oxygen-derived free radicals 73
oxygen tension, transcutaneous 35, 60, 72, 99, 101, 104

pancreas and kidney transplantation, combined (CPKT) 81
papillas 8
paraffin oil 3, 36, 55, 63
paralysis of the leg 93
peak capillary blood cell velocity (pCBV) 22, 67
peak flow, time to 79
percutaneous transluminal angioplasty (PTA) 160
perfusion
 – heterogeneity 118
 – homogeneity 46, 69, 71, 130
 – microvascular 69, 70
periocapillary halo 31, 32, 38
pericytes 78, 88
peripheral arterial occlusive disease (PAOD) 63–65
 – of the arm 67
 – basic classifications of morphological changes 64
 – candle-light phenomenon 73
 – of the leg 67
 – permeability 71
 – and sympathetic blockade 160
peripheral vascular resistance 153
permeability
 – diabetes 82–88
 – after cold injury 151
 – evaluation of 58
 – lymphatic capillary of 43, 73, 78, 82, 99, 130
 – scleroderma 130–134
 – venous disease 98
pharmacological agents 155–161
phlebedema 46, 93
Pick-Herxheimer's disease 151
pigmented network 8

pindolol 156, 158
plasma gaps 11, 15
plasma layer 38, 39, 45, 134, 135
platinum cathode 61
polycythemia 144
 – secondary 145
 – vera 144
polyol-inositol 78
postocclusive reactive hyperemia (PRH) 20–22
postthrombotic state 193
preeclampsia 152–153
pregnancy 152, 153
prelymphatic channels 54
pressure
 – interstitial 99
 – intralymphatic 113
 – ratio 71
Prinzmetal's angina 115
probe
 – triple 61
 – combined 61
progressive systemic sclerosis 121–137
prostanoids 156
proteins, vessel wall 78
proteoglycans 78
purpura 139

radioisotopes
 – labeled 101
Raynaud's phenomenon 5
 – differential diagnosis 139, 141
 – primary 115–117
 – secondary 121–137
 – and vibration 139
reactivity, microvascular 68, 81, 82
recording system 11
red cell column 38, 45, 135
reflex, veno-arteriolar 81
reflux, cutaneous 103, 111
Rendu-Osler-Weber's disease 148–150
reperfusion injury 73
rest pain 71
resting capillary blood cell velocity (rCBV) 18, 22
 – after placebo 155
 – after nifedipine 155
retina, fluorescence angiography of 31
retinopathy 137
 – diabetic 81, 82, 88
retrograde motion, in collectors/precollectors 103
rheology 82, 116
rheumatoid arthritis 138

schizophrenia 153
sclerodactyly 124
scleroderma 38, 99, 121ff.

Subject Index

– CREST variant of 124
– microaneurysms 137
– microangiopathy of 124
– microvascular patterns 123
– prevalence of 124
– transcapillary diffusion 130
– teleangiectasic form of 148
"shock position" 54
shunting, arterio-venous 80, 82, 99
sickle-cell disease 153
Sjögren's syndrome 124
skin surface 2
– flow velocity 79
– induration 93
– ischemia 69
– necrosis 63, 66, 95
– temperature 19, 36, 50, 67, 80
sorbinil 88
spatial correlation 16
spectral transmission, characteristics of ICG 32, 33
spontaneous fluorescence 39
subpapillary vascular plexus 5
surgery, reconstructive arterial 73, 159, 160
systolic blood pressure (SBP) 65
stimulation, spinal cord 161
streptokinase 120

teleangiectasias 122, 123
– hereditary 148
temperature
– control 36
– measurements 12
– skin 49, 67
temporal correlation 16
terbutaline 73
test signal generator 43
thermistors 10
thrombectomy 160
thrombolysis, local 160
thrombosis, microvascular 97, 98, 104
time to peak capillary blood cell velocity (tpCBV) 22
toes 56, 63
tongue 3, 8, 148
total peripheral resistance (TPR) 147
tracers, radioactive 88
transplantation 81, 82
trauma 153

ulcer, venous 101, 105
ulceration, digital 124
urticaria 32

varicous veins 93
vascular plexus, subpapillary 153

vasoconstriction 45
– reflex 69
vasodilatation, maximal 60, 82
vasomotion 69
vasospasms 115, 116, 121, 125, 150
vasospastic
– diseases 115–121
– phenomenon 156
velocity values 18
venous leg ulcers 95, 101, 105
venous insufficiency 38, 60, 93–106
– deep vein (DVI) 94
– incompetent perforators 92
venular limb 5
venules 73, 79, 88
vibration disease 124, 139
video
– camera 10
– fluorescence microscopy 34–44
– monitoring 10
– recording 2
vinblastine 139
viscosity, blood 153
vitreous, in diabetics 78, 82, 88
von Willebrand factor 78

wedge 3
white cell, trapping 97, 98, 104